Get Thr

MRCGP

Barts and T
Queen Mary's School of M

WHITECHAPEL LIBRARY
0.

Books

Get Through
MRCGP: Hot Topics

Una Coales MD FRCS FRCSOTO DRCOG DFFP MRCGP
GP, London, UK

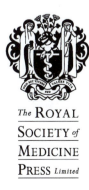

The ROYAL
SOCIETY *of*
MEDICINE
PRESS *Limited*

© 2005 Royal Society of Medicine Ltd

Reprinted 2006

Published by the Royal Society of Medicine Press Ltd
1 Wimpole Street, London W1G 0AE, UK
Tel: +44 (0)20 7290 2921
Fax: +44 (0)20 7290 2929
Email: publishing@rsm.ac.uk
Website: www.rsmpress.co.uk

British Library Cataloguing in Publication Data
A catalogue record for this book is available from the British Library

ISBN: 1-85315-680-9

Distribution in Europe and Rest of the World:

Marston Book Services Ltd
PO Box 269
Abingdon
Oxon OX14 4YN, UK
Tel: +44 (0)1235 465500
Fax: +44 (0)1235 465555
Email: direct.order@marston.co.uk

Distribution in USA and Canada:

Royal Society of Medicine Press Ltd
c/o Jamco Distribution Inc
1401 Lakeway Drive
Lewisville, TX 75057, USA
Tel: +1 800 538 1287
Fax: +1 972 353 1303
Email: jamco@majors.com

Distribution in Australia and New Zealand:

Elsevier Australia
30-52 Smidmore Street
Marrikville NSW 2204, Australia
Tel: +61 2 9517 8999
Fax: +61 2 9517 2249
Email: service@elsevier.com.au

Phototypeset by Saxon Graphics Ltd, Derby
Printed in the UK by Bell & Bain Ltd, Glasgow

Contents

Preface

This book accompanies both *Get Through MRCGP: New MCQ Module* and *Get Through MRCGP: Oral and Video Modules*. Hot topics need updating frequently. This book contains the most up-to-date clinical guidelines (NICE, SIGN, BTS, Royal Colleges, etc.) for the management of chronic diseases, including the 2004 BTS/NICE guidelines for COPD, dyspepsia and the 2004 BHS guidelines for hypertension. Also included is an A to Z of all hot topics that have been asked in recent examination modules. Further topics include the DVLA Guidelines for Fitness to Drive (amended in January 2004), welfare benefits, child development and statistics. All topics are presented in an easy-to-read outline format for ease of memorisation. Sources for the material covered include the weekly *British Medical Journal*, the weekly *Doctor* magazines, the Oxford Handbook Series, the BNF and websites for all current government and college guidelines. This book is therefore a culmination of several months spent reading and summarising hot topics.

Una Coales
ufcmd@aol.com

Recommended texts and references

Birtwhistle J. *et al.* (2002) *Oxford Handbook of General Practice*. Oxford University Press, Oxford.

British Thoracic Society Guidelines and Scottish Intercollegiate Guidelines Network (2003) *Thorax* 58(Suppl I): I1–I69.

British Thoracic Society Guidelines and National Institute for Clinical Excellence (2004) *Chronic obstructive pulmonary disease*, National Institute for Clinical Excellence, London.

Coales U. (2003) *Get Through MRCGP: New MCQ Module*, The Royal Society of Medicine Press, London.

Coales U. (2004) *Get Through MRCGP: Oral and Video Modules*. The Royal Society of Medicine Press, London.

Collier J.A.B. *et al.* (2003) *Oxford Handbook of Clinical Specialties*, 6th edn. Oxford University Press, Oxford.

Davies T. *et al.* (1998) *ABC of Mental Health*, 1st edn. BMJ Books, London.

Department of Health (1999) *Drug Misuse and Dependence – Guidelines on Clinical Management*. HMSO, London.

Drivers Medical Group, DVLA (2004) *Fitness to Drive Guidelines*. DVLA, Swansea.

Glasier A. *et al.* (2000) *Handbook of Family Planning and Reproductive Healthcare*, 4th edn. Churchill Livingstone, London.

Health and Safety Commission (1999) *Management of Health and Safety at Work. Approved Code of Practice and Guidance*. HSE Books, Sudbury, Suffolk.

Hope R.A. *et al.* (2001) *Oxford Handbook of Clinical Medicine*, 5th edn. Oxford University Press, Oxford.

Neighbour R. (2002) *The Inner Consultation*. Librapharm, Newbury, Berkshire.

Palmer K.T. (2001) *Notes for the MRCGP*, 3rd edn. Blackwell Science, Oxford.

Royal Pharmaceutical Society of Great Britain (2004) *British National Formulary*. British Medical Association, London.

McLatchie G.R. (2001) *Oxford Handbook of Clinical Surgery*, 2nd edn. Oxford University Press, Oxford.

Roland N.J. *et al.* (2000) *Key Topics in Otolaryngology*, 2nd edn. BIOS Scientific Publishers, Oxford.

Abbreviations

AC	air conduction
ACE	angiotensin-converting enzyme
APD	relative afferent pupillary defect
ATIIR	angiotensin II receptor antagonist
BCC	basal cell carcinoma
BDR	background retinopathy
BHS	British Hypertension Society
BMI	body mass index
BP	blood pressure
BTS	British Thoracic Society
CA	carcinoma
CABG	coronary artery bypass grafting
CDT	community drug team
CHD	coronary heart disease
CN	cranial nerve
COAD	coronary obstructive airways disease
COPD	coronary obstructive pulmonary disease
CPA	costophrenic angle
CRC	colorectal cancer
CRP	C-reactive protein
CT	computed tomography
CV	cardiovascular
CVA	cerebrovascular accident
DBP	diastolic blood pressure
DM	diabetes mellitus
DVT	deep vein thrombosis
EAC	external auditory canal
EAM	external auditory meatus
EBV	Epstein–Barr virus
ECG	electrocardiogram, -graphy
ENT	ear, nose and throat
EOMI	extra-ocular movements intact
ESR	erythrocyte sedimentation rate
EUA	examination under anaesthesia
FB	foreign body
FBC	full blood count
FESS	functional endoscopic sinus surgery
FEV_1	forced expiratory volume in 1 second
FH	family history
FNE	fine needle exam
GA	general anaesthesia
GI	gastrointestinal
GN	glomerulonephritis
Hb	haemoglobin
HDL	high density lipoprotein
HIV	human immunodeficiency virus
HNPCC	hereditary non-polyposis colorectal cancer
HRT	hormone replacement therapy
HSV	herpes simplex virus

HVS	high vaginal swab
I+D	incision and drainage
IDDM	insulin-dependent diabetes mellitus
IOP	intraocular pressure
IVIs	intravenous fluid infusion
LA	local anaesthesia
LABA	long-acting beta-agonist
LBP	low blood pressure
LDL	low density lipoprotein
LFT	liver function tests
LMN	lower motor neuron
LMP	last menstrual period
LOC	loss of consciousness
LVEF	left ventricular ejection fraction
LVF	left ventricular failure
MCP	metacarpophalangeal
MDI	metered dose inhaler
MI	myocardial infarction
MRC	Medical Research Council
MRI	magnetic resonance imaging
MSU	mid-stream urine
MTP	metatarsophalangeal
MUA	manipulation under anaesthesia
MVA	motor vehicle accident
NLP	neuro-linguistic programming
NICE	National Institute of Clinical Excellence
NIDDM	non-insulin-dependent diabetes mellitus
NPV	negative predictive value
NSAIDs	non-steroidal anti-inflammatory drugs
N/V	nausea/vomiting
N/V/D	nausea/vomiting/diarrhoea
OCD	obsessive-compulsive disorder
OE	on examination
OM	otitis media
OPC	outpatient clinic
PCP	*Pneumocystis carinii* pneumonia
PCT	primary care trust
PD	Parkinson's disease
PDP	personal development plan
PE	pulmonary embolism
PEF	peak exploratory flow
PFM	peak flow meter
PID	pelvic inflammatory disease
PIP	proximal interphalangeal
PNS	post-nasal space
PPI	proton pump inhibitor
PPV	positive predictive value
PR	per rectum
PSA	prostate specific antigen
PTA	pure tone audiogram
PUVA	ultraviolet A
PV	per vagina

px	prescription
RAPD	relative afferent pupillary defect
RBBB	right bundle branch block
RCT	randomised controlled trial
RF	risk factor
SBP	systolic blood pressure
SCC	squamous cell carcinoma
SIGN	Scottish Intercollegiate Guidelines Network
SLR	straight leg raise
SNHL	sensorineural hearing loss
SOB	short of breath
SSRIs	selective serotonin reuptake inhibitors
STD	sexually transmitted disease
TB	tuberculosis
TC	total cholesterol
TFT	thyroid function test
TG	triglycerides
TIA	transient ischaemic attack
TM	tympanic membrane
tx	treatment
UGI	upper gastrointestinal
UPSI	unprotected sexual intercourse
UTI	urinary tract infection
URT	upper respiratory tract
URTI	upper respiratory tract infection
U/S	ultrasound
UVB	ultraviolet B
UVPPP	uvulopalatopharyngoplasty
VA	visual acuity
WHO	World Health Organization

Acne Case Management

This is a common ailment among teenagers.

Case scenario 1

A 14-year-old female presents with persistent acne on the forehead. Management involves triple therapy consisting of Erythroped (erythromycin), Differin (adapalene) cream topically to the face and Dianette (co-cyprindiol) od. This form of therapy should be taken consistently for at least 3 months. Erythroped is a paediatric tablet without the side-effects of nausea and vomiting.

Explain that Dianette may be associated with side-effects such as headache and breast tenderness. The patient is then weaned off Erythroped from bd for 1 month to od for 1 month and then stopped. If there have been no flares, stop the Dianette and leave the Differin cream as prophylaxis.

Roaccutane (isotretinoin) is discouraged, as the drug is not well tolerated. Side-effects include dry skin, muscle aches and pains and flu-like symptoms. However it prevents acne for one year.

Case scenario 2

A 13-year-old female presents with acne or widespread maculopapular rash with postinflammatory changes over her back, arms and chest. She does not tolerate Erythroped (erythromycin).

Try triple therapy with trimethoprim 200 mg bd, Dianette (co-cyprindiol) and Differin (adapalene) gel to be applied thinly od. If she does not tolerate trimethoprim, try Minocin MR (minocycline).

Analgaesia

This is a favourite topic for the MRCGP MCQ module.

Bone pain from metastases   NSAID

Dysmenorrhoea (fibroids)   mefenamic acid

Mechanical back pain   paracetamol

Migraine   sumatriptan ($5HT_1$ agonist) if simple analgaesia fails; not ergot alkaloids

Postherpetic neuralgia   amitriptyline (first-line); gabapentin (second-line)

Renal colic   diclofenac IM

Sickle cell crisis   morphine; not pethidine which can precipitate fits

Trigeminal neuralgia   carbamazepine

Antibiotics

Amoxicillin acute bronchitis; acute exacerbation of COPD; acute otitis media; bacteriocidal; community-acquired pneumonia; sinusitis; cellulitis

Benzylpenicillin IV suspected meningitis (*Neisseria meningitidis*) – 1200 mg for adults and children > 10 years old; 600 mg for children 1–9 years old; 300 mg for babies < 1 year old.

Ciprofloxacin acute pyelonephritis or use co-amoxiclav; gonorrhoea – treat with ciprofloxacin 500 mg STAT or if pregnant, give amoxicillin 3 g + probencid 1 g oral STAT and test for cure; PID (ciprofloxacin 500 mg STAT + doxycycline 100 mg bd for 2 weeks + metronidazole 400 mg bd for 5 days)

Co-amoxiclavulanic acid human bites (URT aerobes + anaerobes); animal bites (*Pasteurella multicoda, Capnocytophagia canimorsus*, anaerobes, call the Communicable Diseases Surveillance Centre (CCDC) for rabies, check tetanus status)

Doxycycline *Chlamydia trachomatis* 100 mg bd for 1 week or azithromycin 1 g STAT; test for cure in 1 month for chlamydia

Erythromycin atypical pneumonia; bacteriostatic; penicillin allergy; clarithromycin to non-responders

Flucloxacillin folliculitis (*Staph. aureus* + Gram-negative organism); impetigo (*Staph. aureus, Strep. pyogenes*); infected wounds

Metronidazole bacterial vaginosis (gardnerella – Gram-negative anaerobe); Aci-Gel for recurrent cases; *Trichomonas vaginalis* treat with 400 mg bd for 5 days

Oxytetracycline 500 mg bd for acne; second-line or pregnant: erythromycin 500 mg bd

Phenoxymethylpenicillin   + flucloxacillin for cellulitis (*Staph. aureus, Strep. pyogenes*); acute tonsillitis

Trimethoprim   uncomplicated UTI treat with 200 mg bd for 3 days; alternative nitrofurantoin 50 mg 6 hourly; if pregnant treat with cefadroxil 500 mg bd

Anxiety

Anxiety may be subdivided into seven categories:

1. OCD (obsessive–compulsive disorder):

- The obsessions are one's own thoughts, repetitive in nature, intrusive and causing distress (ego–dystonic).
- The patient acknowledges that these are irrational silly thoughts and attempts to resist the thoughts.
- The treatment for OCD is with SSRIs such as clomipramine or fluoxetine (at a higher dose than recommended for depression).

2. Phobias:

- May be subdivided again into simple, social and agoraphobia. A phobia is a fear to one stimulus and is manifested by avoidance and anticipatory anxiety.
- Simple phobia is treated with behavioural therapy.
- Social phobia is treated with an SSRI such as fluoxetine. Agoraphobia may coexist with a panic disorder.

3. Panic disorder:

- Is severe, acute onset anxiety and is manifested by autonomic symptoms, cognitive symptoms (fear of dying or collapse) and muscular symptoms (tightening).
- The treatment is with both cognitive behavioural therapy and SSRI medication. Be wary of paroxetine, which is associated with a discontinuation syndrome with 'panic anxiety'. Beta-blockers are not recommended.

4. Generalised anxiety disorder:

- Is a free-floating anxiety.
- The patient is constantly on edge with a general feeling of discomfort.
- The recommended treatment is with SSRIs.

5. Adjustment disorders:

- Occur as a result of life events such as grief or death. SSRIs are not of value here.

6. Post-traumatic stress disorder:

- Is anxiety brought on by an event outside the realms of normal trauma (rape, severe mugging) and manifests itself by recurrent nightmares, flashbacks, avoidance.

- Recommended treatment is with SSRIs and a referral to trauma services.

7. Somatoform disorder:

- Presents with physical symptoms. There are two forms of somatoform disorders – somatisation and hypochondriacal.

- Somatisation is more common in women and lasts for less than 6 months. The patient may ask for relief of his or her symptoms with tablets.

- Hypochondriacal patients are often in their late thirties or forties and will ask for confirmation of one or two disease processes with investigations such as an MR scan. The latter occurs in men and women in equal ratio.

- The motive in patients with factitious disorder or Münchausen's syndrome is to be ill. They are addicted to hospitals and will resort to changing their names, hospitals, deceiving and undergoing multiple unnecessary operations.

8. Malingering:

- Patients fabricate symptoms for an ulterior motive such as sick notes and benefits.

9. Hysteria:

- Acute stress followed by a physical symptom, which cannot be explained neurologically. An example of this would be acute onset of left leg paralysis. The patient is unable to cope with anxiety and develops a dissociative symptom.

Asthma Case Management

Asthma is the most common cause of wheeze, nocturnal cough, and chronic productive cough in children.

Case scenario

A 10-year-old girl presents complaining of a 4-month history of productive cough that has failed three courses of antibiotic treatment. The cough is worse at night and the sputum clear.

Management:

1. Take a pertinent history of the presenting complaint:
   - Can she hear any wheezing?
   - Does she wheeze with exercise?
   - Does she have any food allergies?
   - Does she suffer from eczema or hayfever?
   - Does she cough more at night?

2. Ask about her past history:
   - Ask questions regarding her birth and school.
   - Is she up to date with her immunisations?
   - Has she had her BCG injection?
   - How are her siblings?
   - Is there a family history of asthma or allergies?
   - What is the occupation of both parents?
   - Are there any pets in the house or does she come into contact with any pets?
   - Is her bedroom carpeted?

3. Perform a physical examination:
   - Check her fingers for clubbing.
   - Palpate her neck for lymph nodes.
   - Auscultate her chest both anteriorly and posteriorly and ask her to cough.
   - Examine her arms and legs for any signs of eczema.

4. Demonstrate the use of a peak-flow meter. Offer the child a peak-flow meter and measure her peak flow. Record the best of three attempts and compare the reading with a standardised chart.

5. Administer one puff of Ventolin (salbutamol) inhaler through a spacer and ask the patient to pant briskly to absorb the Ventolin. Repeat three more times and have the child sit and rest.

6. Repeat the peak flow. Her performance should markedly improve. Spirometry is a better marker of lung function but is only offered in a paediatric chest clinic.

7. Ask the child to supply sputum in a specimen pot for microscopy, culture and sensitivities.

8. Arrange for a chest x-ray to exclude bronchiectasis, pneumonia and tuberculosis.

9. Prescribe a 6-week trial course of Flixotide bd (fluticasone propionate, a steroid inhaler) and Ventolin prn 4 hourly.

10. Ensure the parent makes a follow-up appointment in 6 weeks' time to assess progress.

11. If the child does suffer from allergies, the child may be referred to the paediatric chest outpatient clinic or the ENT department for skin prick allergy testing.

Asthma Management in Adults

(British Thoracic Society and SIGN 2003)

Step	Reliever	Additional therapies		Further advice/therapy
1 Mild intermittent	Inhaled short-acting β_2-agonist prn			Review if > 10–12 puffs/day
2 Regular preventer	Inhaled short-acting β_2-agonist prn	Add inhaled steroid 200–800 μg/day		Titrate to lowest effective dose. Usual starting dose 400 μg/day. Divide dose twice daily and then once daily when controlled
3 Add on therapy	Inhaled short-acting β_2-agonist prn	Inhaled steroid 200–800 μg/day	Add inhaled LABA	Continue LABA. Increase steroid to 800 μg, if still poorly controlled. If no response to LABA, stop LABA, increase steroid to 800 μg/day. Consider adding fourth drug (leukotriene receptor antagonists, slow release β_2-agonist tablets of theophylline).
4 Persistent poor control	Inhaled short-acting β_2-agonist prn	Inhaled steroid 800 μg/day	Inhaled LABA (unless no effect)	Consider trials of increased steroids to 2000 μg. Consider trials of fourth drug. Consider referral to specialist
5 Continuous or frequent oral steroids	Inhaled short-acting β_2-agonist prn	High dose inhaled steroid 2000 μg/day	Add oral steroids at lowest effective dose	Consider other treatments to minimise oral steroids. Refer to specialist

Aims: Minimise symptoms during day and night.
Minimise need for reliever.
No exacerbations.
No physical activity limitation.
Normal lung function (FEV$_1$ +/or PEF > 80%
predicted or best).

Treatment: Start treatment at level appropriate to asthma
severity.
Step up treatment as required (prior to starting
new therapy, recheck compliance, inhaler
technique and remove trigger factors; if trials of
add-on therapies are ineffective, cease; if trials of
increased steroids are ineffective, return to original
dose).
Step down treatment levels when control
achieved. Review regularly.

Steroid therapy: Refers to beclomethasone dipropionate via an
MDI.
Inhaled steroids advised after exacerbations,
nocturnal asthma, impaired lung function or with
more than once daily β_2-agonist.
20–50% dose reduction every 3 months.
Systemic side-effects with long-term or frequent
oral steroids – monitor BP, review for signs of
diabetes and osteoporosis. In children, monitor
growth, check for signs of adrenal suppression and
screen for cataracts.

Asthma Management in Children
British Thoracic Society and SIGN 2003

Children under 5 years

Step	Reliever	Additional therapies		Further advice/therapy
1	Inhaled short-acting β_2-agonist prn			Review if high usage
2	Inhaled short-acting β_2-agonist prn	Add inhaled steroid (200–400 μg/day) or add other preventer (leukotriene receptor antagonists) if steroids cannot be used		Usual starting dose 200 μg/day divided twice daily
3	Inhaled short-acting β_2-agonist prn	Inhaled steroid (200–400 μg/day).	Consider trial of leukotriene receptor antagonists. If < 2 years old, consider proceed to step 4	
4	Inhaled short-acting β_2-agonist prn	Inhaled steroid (400 μ/day)		Refer to paediatric specialist

Children aged 5–12 years

Step	Reliever	Additional therapies		Further advice/therapy
1 Mild intermittent	Inhaled short-acting β_2-agonist prn			Review if high usage
2 Regular preventer	Inhaled short-acting β_2-agonist prn	Add inhaled steroid (200–400 µg/day) or add other preventer (leukotriene receptor antagonists) if steroids cannot be used		Usual starting dose 200 µg/day divided twice daily
3 Add-on therapy	Inhaled short-acting β_2-agonist prn	Inhaled steroid (200–400 µg/day).	Add LABA	Continue LABA. Increase steroid to 400 µg/day, if still poorly controlled and stop LABA if no response to LABA. Consider adding fourth drug (leukotriene receptor antagonists, theophylline)
4 Persistent poor control	Inhaled short-acting β_2-agonist prn	Inhaled steroid (400 µ/day).	Inhaled LABA	Consider trials of increased steroids and referral to specialist
5 Continuous or frequent use of oral steroids	Inhaled short-acting β_2-agonist prn	Inhaled steroid (800 µ/day).	Use oral steroids at lowest dose	Refer to paediatric specialist

Back Pain

Clinical Guidelines for the Management of Acute Low Back Pain: Royal College of General Practitioners 1999

1. Simple backache (non-specific low back pain) – 90%

- 20–55 years old.
- Lumbosacral, buttocks and thigh.
- 'Mechanical' pain – varies with physical activity and time.
- Well patient.
- Specialist referral is not required.
- X-rays are not routinely indicated, as soft tissue injuries cannot be detected on x-ray or MRI. Back x-rays have 120 times the radiation of a chest x-ray.
- 90% recover within 6 weeks.
- Consider psychosocial factors (yellow flags).
- Prescribe regular analgaesia – start with paracetamol, may then substitute NSAIDs and then codydramol or coproxamol. Finally consider adding a short course of a muscle relaxant such as baclofen or diazepam.
- Avoid narcotics.
- Do not recommend bedrest. Bedrest for 2–7 days is worse than placebo or ordinary activity.
- Advise patients to stay active and resume normal daily activities.
- Consider manipulative treatment within the first 6 weeks for patients who are failing to return to normal activities.
- Refer for reactivation/rehabilitation if back pain persists more than 6 weeks.

2. Nerve root pain – < 5%

- Specialist referral is not generally required within the first 4 weeks, provided resolving.
- Absent ankle jerk or numbness.
- Unilateral leg pain worse than LBP.
- Pain radiates to foot or toes.
- Pain is worse after coughing.
- Numbness and paraesthesia are in the same direction.

- Nerve irritation signs – reduced SLR reproduces leg pain.
- Localised neurological signs – limited to one nerve root.
- 50% recover spontaneously from acute attack within 6 weeks.
- Full recovery expected but recurrence possible.

3. Red flags for potentially serious spinal pathology (urgent referral < 4 weeks)

- Presentation under age 20 or over age 55.
- Constant, progressive, non-mechanical pain.
- Violent trauma.
- Past history of CA, drug abuse, HIV or systemic steroids.
- Persistent severe restriction of lumbar flexion.
- Structural deformity.
- Thoracic pain.
- Systemically unwell, weight loss.
- Widespread neurology.
- Note: MRI has a high false positive rate and is abnormal on everyone > 30 years who shows disk protrusion. By age 50, we all have lumbar spondylosis.

4. Cauda equina syndrome (immediate referral)

- Gait disturbance.
- Saddle anaesthesia.
- Sphincter disturbance.

5. Yellow flags (psychosocial risk factors): Kendall et al 1997

- A belief that back pain is harmful or potentially severely disabling.
- Fear-avoidance behaviour and reduced activity levels. Have you had time off work in the past with back pain? When do you think you will return to work?
- Tendency to low mood and withdrawal from social interaction.
- Expectation of passive treatment(s) rather than a belief that active participation will help.
- Patients are at risk of chronic low back pain and poor prognosis.
- Consider specialised psychological referrals for those with psychopathology.

6. Vertebral fractures – < 5%

- Assess risk factors such as early menopause, previous fracture, prolonged steroids.

7. Inflammatory conditions – 1%

- i.e. Ankylosing spondylitis (early twenties, male, with morning stiffness and pain or after sitting for 1 hour watching television).

8. Malignancy/infection – < 1%

- Paget's disease is painless.
- Metastatic pain is continuous, unremitting, throbbing nocturnal pain.

Benefits (Welfare)

1. Free prescriptions

< 16 years old

16–18 year olds in full-time education

60 years old or over

pregnant or you have had a baby in the last year (FP92)

medical exemptions (Addison's disease, diabetes mellitus, epilepsy, fistulae, hypopituitarism, myasthaenia gravis, myxoedema)

war or MoD pensioner

entitled to a prepayment certificate (FP96)

NHS low income scheme (HC2 certificate)

receiving benefits from income support, family credit, DWA (Disability Work Allowance), Job-seeker's Allowance

2. Disability and handicap

Attendance Allowance

> 65 years, severe mental or physical disability;
lasting > 6 months, daycare or day + night rate, tax free, non-means tested; supervision to prevent injury and help required to perform bodily functions

Disability Living Allowance

> 5 years old and < 65 years old; requires care;
+ immobility, (unable to walk) for 3 months, lasting > 6 months

Disability Working Allowance

low income > 16 years old, 16 hours/week, receiving one of the disability allowances; tax-free BUT income-related and means-tested

Incapacity Benefit	paid at three rates (short-term up to 28 weeks at lower rate, higher rate from 28 weeks to 1 year, long-term rate after 1 year); if one is unfit to work on medical grounds for > 28 weeks and has paid NI contributions (issue med 4 after 28 weeks)
Invalid Care Allowance	carers looking after dependants, handicapped; 16–64 years; 35 hours/week as carer, < £50/week earnings; dependant on Attendance Allowance, Disability Living Allowance or Constant Attendance Allowance
Severe Disability Allowance	80% disabled or unable to work under twentieth birthday; no NI contributions; unable to work for > 28 weeks, 16–65 years

3. Low income and other benefits

Child Benefit	< 16 years old, tax free; not means tested
Disabled Person's Tax Credit	work > 16 hours/week; means tested
Incapacity Benefit	not entitled to statutory sick pay; self-employed
Income Support	18 years old over, working < 16 hours/week; means tested; savings £3000 or less
Maternity Incapacity Benefit	in last 6 weeks and 2 weeks postpartum
Social Fund payments	budget loan; crisis loan; community care grant; cold weather payments, funeral expenses; maternity grant
Statutory Maternity Allowance	worked at least 26 weeks of 66 weeks prior to due date and paid NI for 8 weeks prior. 18 weeks' pay; apply for MATB1 > 20/40
Statutory Sick Pay	16–65 years old; unable to work between 4 days and 28 weeks

Visually handicapped

< 3/60 blind, < 6/60 partially sighted,
cheaper TV licence, parking + travel fare concessions

Deafness

Social Services arrange doorbells, flashing alarms, travel concessions

Working Family's Tax Credit

work > 16 hours/week with children;
means tested

Cancer

Urgent referrals < 2 / week

Breast cancer:

- A discrete lump in a patient over 25 years.

- Signs suggestive of cancer: acquired skin dimpling, acquired unilateral nipple inversion, persisting unilateral nipple inversion, ulceration or eczema.

- Blood-stained nipple discharge at any age associated with a mass.

- Localised persisting nodularity in a patient over 30 years.

- Persisting signs of sepsis in a non-lactating breast.

- Note: Refer to family history clinic for breast cancer in an immediate relative, i.e. sister, mother, aunt or maternal grandmother with single case diagnosis under age 40, two cases under age 50, three cases at any age when diagnosed or an association of breast and ovarian cancer in an individual or family member.

Skin cancer:

- Melanoma (pigmented lesion with one of the following features):
  - change in colour
  - change in shape
  - increase in size (usually $\geq$ 5 mm at diagnosis)
  - inflammation
  - irregular borders
  - mixed colour
  - ulceration.

- Squamous cell carcinoma:
  - diagnosed on biopsy in general practice surgery
  - non-healing, indurated, slow-growing (over 1–2 months) lesions on face, scalp or back of hand
  - transplant patients who develop new or growing cutaneous lesions.

Upper GI cancer:

- Dysphagia.
- Dyspepsia with one of the following risk factors:
  - continuous symptoms since onset in a patient ≥ 55 years
  - family history of upper GI cancer in at least two first-degree relatives
  - known dysplasia, atrophic gastritis, intestinal metaplasia
  - new onset (< 1 year) in a patient ≥ 55 years
  - peptic ulcer surgery > 20 years ago
  - pernicious anaemia
  - proven anaemia
  - vomiting
  - weight loss.
- Jaundice.
- Upper abdominal mass.

Urological cancer:

- Macroscopic haematuria.
- Microscopic haematuria in adults > 50 years.
- Palpable renal masses.
- PSA > 20 ng/ml in men with a clinically malignant prostate or bone pain.
- Solid renal masses found on imaging.
- Suspected penile cancer.
- Swellings in the body of the testis.

SIGN Management of Colorectal Cancer – National Clinical Guidelines, March 2003

Prevention:

- Eat five portions of fruit and vegetables each day.
- HRT use is not preventative.
- Maintain BMI ≤ 25 kg/m².
- Take 30 minutes of exercise a day.

Screening of patients at high risk:

- Inflammatory bowel disease:
  - annual colonoscopy for disease of 20 years' duration or with indeterminate dysplasia
  - 3-yearly colonoscopy with biopsies for left-sided colitis or pancolitis for 10 years
  - colectomy for high grade dysplasia and consider for low grade also.
- Following colonoscopic removal of adenomatous polyps:
  - mandatory follow-up colonosopy
  - if one or two adenomas > 1 cm are found, repeat colonoscopy at 5 years
  - if three adenomas are found or at least one > 1 cm or with severe dysplasia, perform 3-yearly colonoscopies.
- High-risk family history of colorectal cancer:
  - HNPCC gene carriers
  - three family members with CRC
  - two family members with CRC + one with endometrial cancer in at least two generations
  - offer 2-yearly colonoscopy
  - offer 2-yearly UGI endoscopy
  - discuss screening for endometrial and ovarian CA.

Urgent referral guidelines:

- All patients with iron-deficiency anaemia (Hb < 11 g/dl in men and < 10 g/dl in postmenopausal women) who do not have an overt cause.
- Patients > 50 years who have had one of the following symptoms for 6 weeks:
  - intestinal obstruction
  - palpable abdominal or rectal mass
  - rectal bleeding with a change in bowel habit to increased frequency or looseness
  - rectal bleeding without anal symptoms.

Cervical Smear

Screening:

- Offered at 3-yearly or 5-yearly intervals (depending on local health authority).
- Offered to women between the ages of 20 and 64.
- According to an audit conducted by the Cancer Research UK NHS Cervical Screening Programme, results show that women under the age of 25 should not be screened; it recommmends 3-yearly screening for women between 25 and 49, and 5-yearly screening for women between 50 and 64.
- In the USA, cervical screening occurs at 2-yearly intervals as studies show cervical cancers are missed if screened at later intervals.

Borderline atypia or dyskaryosis (borderline CIN):

- Repeat smear at 6 months.
- Refer for colposcopy if there are two or three borderline smears at 6-monthly intervals.

Mild dyskaryosis (Grade 1 CIN):

- Check local policy.
- Contentious whether to repeat smear at 6 months or refer immediately for colposcopy as there is a 30% risk of the patient already having CIN 2 or 3 changes.

Moderate and severe dyskaryosis (Grades 2 and 3 CIN):

- Refer immediately for colposcopy.
- According to a study in New Zealand one third of untreated women with CIN 3 developed cervical cancer over a 20-year period.

Child Development Milestones

6 weeks	Follows objects 1 m away, grasp, Moro, smiles, startles
12 weeks	Turns head to sounds on the same level with the ear
6 months	Person preference, sits with support, transfers cube hand to hand, crude touch
7 months	Feeds self a biscuit, turns head to sound below the level of the ear
8 months	Sits without support
9 months	Afraid of strangers, crawls on abdomen, pincer grasp
12 months	Uses two to three words, walks with one hand held
18 months	Uses 10–12 words, asks for potty, uses spoon, can construct a three- or four-cube tower, jumps with both feet
2 years	Can construct a six- or seven-cube tower, kicks a ball, plays with children alongside
2.5–3 years	Scribbles
3 years	Knows age and sex, joins three words into a sentence, plays with other children, ascends with one foot per step but descends with two feet per step, knows two colours
4 years	Knows first and last name, can copy a circle, can copy a cross, catch a ball, rides a tricycle
5 years	Counts 10–12 objects, knows three or four colours, hops on one foot, has own set of friends

Childhood Illnesses

Chickenpox

Incubation 14–16 days; short or no interval between onset and rash. Rash lesion of different stages: spots in crops → macule → papule → vesicle. Complications: eczema herpeticum, encephalitis, pneumonia.

Erythema infectiosum (parvovirus, fifth disease)

Mild fever, slapped cheek (erythematous maculopapular rash), reticular lacy rash on trunk and limbs, duration 4–7 days.

Hand, foot and mouth disease (Coxsackie virus)

Mild fever, oral blisters, red vesicles on palms and soles. Duration: 4–7 days.

Measles

Incubation 10–14 days; early – coryzal symptoms, conjunctivitis, fever; later – buccal Koplik spots, 4 days between onset and florid maculopapular rash on face, behind ear, chest. Complications: bronchopneumonia, encephalitis, subacute sclerosing panencephalitis. Duration: 10 days. Antibiotics for secondary infections.

Mumps

Incubation 16–21 days; fever, malaise, parotid or submandibular gland enlargement. Complications: aseptic meningitis, epididymo-orchitis, pancreatitis.

Roseola infantum

Occurs in childen less than 2 years of age; fever, sore throat, after 3–4 days faint erythematous macular rash; when fever goes, much better. Duration: 4–7 days.

Rubella/German measles

Incubation 14–21 days; mild, suboccipital lymph nodes, short or no interval between disease onset and pink macular rash; transient rash, occurs commonly in teenagers. Complications: birth defects in pregnancy, arthritis in teens. Duration: 10 days.

Scarlet fever

Incubation 2–4 days; 1–2 day interval; long infectivity period shortened by treatment, scarlet facial flushing, coated strawberry tongue, truncal rash, non-exudative tonsillitis, circumoral pallor. Complications: acute GN, rheumatic fever. prescribe penicillin for 10 days.

Typhoid   Incubation 3 days to 3 weeks. 7–14 days
between onset and rash; malaise, fever, cough,
nose bleeds, bruising, truncal rose spots,
splenomegaly. Coma. Adverse reaction to vaccine
increases in those > 35 years old, given 3-yearly

Childhood Immunisations

2, 3, 4 months	Hib–DTP (thigh), polio (oral), Men C (thigh)
12–15 months	MMR (thigh)
Preschool to 4 years	booster MMR (arm), Infantrix (Hib-DTP) arm, oral polio
12 years	BCG if tuberculin negative
14–18 years	Adult dT + polio + Men AC if Men C already given + MMR (if not given)

Cholesterol

Aims

Fasting total cholesterol level < 5 mmol/l

Fasting LDL cholesterol level < 3 mmol/l

Fasting triglyceride level < 2.3 mmol/l

↓

Reduce cholesterol and fat in diet
(3 month trial)

↙   ↘

Cholesterol > 5 mmol/l   normal cholesterol

TG < 2.3 mmol/l   TG > 2.3 mmol/l

↓   ↓

Start statin   Start fibrate

↓   ↓

Review 3 monthly and titrate doses.

↙   ↘

Switch to   Add fibrate if   ↓
stronger statin   TG > 2.3 mmol/l

↓   ↓   ↓

Targets still unmet after 12 months, then refer to lipid clinic

Chronic Obstructive Pulmonary Disease Management

British Thoracic Society/NICE Guidelines 2004

Diagnosis:

- Assess lung function using spirometry
- (FEV_1 < 80% predicted, FEV_1/FVC < 0.7)
- BMI
- MRC dyspnoea score:

Grade Degree of breathlessness related to activity

1	Not troubled by breathlessness except on strenuous activity
2	SOB when walking or hurrying up a slight hill
3	Walks slower than others on level ground or has to stop for breath when walking at own pace
4	Stops for breath after walking 100 m or after a few minutes
5	Too breathless to leave the house

Investigations:

- Chest x-ray
- Haemoglobin to exclude anaemia and polycythaemia

Additional investigations:

- CT scan chest
- ECG
- Echocardiogram
- SaO_2 (severe COAD)
- Serial PFMs showing 20% diurnal variation suggests asthma
- Sputum culture
- Transfer factor for carbon monoxide
- α-1-antitrypsin deficiency if early onset or +FH
- Mild or moderate – assess annually
- Severe – assess twice yearly

Classification:

- Mild (50–80% predicted FEV_1)
- Moderate (30–49%)
- Severe (< 30%)

Consider diagnosis:

- \> 35 years old

- Smoker/ex-smoker

- Symptoms (exertional breathlessness, chronic cough, regular sputum production, frequent winter bronchitis or wheeze)

- No signs of asthma

Treatment for mild to moderate COPD:

Short-acting β_2-agonist or anticholinergic prn

Combined short-acting bronchodilators (β_2-agonist+ anticholinergic)

Long-acting bronchodilator (β_2-agonist or anticholinergic)

↓

One or more bronchodilators (β_2-agonist or anticholinergic)

Treatment for moderate to severe COPD:

One or more bronchodilators (β_2-agonist or anticholinergic)

Long-acting bronchodilator + inhaled steroid (stop if no benefit in 4 weeks)
Inhaled steroids are added to decrease frequency of exacerbations in patients with $FEV_1 \leq 50\%$ predicted who have had two or more exacerbations requiring antibiotics or oral steroids in the past 12 months.

Consider adding theophylline

Oral steroids and/or antibiotics and non-invasive ventilation during exacerbations

Additional supportive measures:

- Encourage smoking cessation

- Pulmonary rehab. if appropriate

- Mucolytic therapy for chronic productive cough

- Non-invasive ventilation for persistent hypercapnic ventilatory failure

- Long-term O_2 therapy (for $PaO2 < 7.3$ kPa and stable or for $PaO2 > 7.3$ kPa but < 8 kPa when stable with secondary symptoms)

- Ambulatory and short burst O_2 should be given as needed
- Address obesity and poor nutrition
- Influenza/pneumococcal vaccination
- Identify and treat depression associated with COPD
- Self-management advice for exacerbations

Specialist referral:

- Diagnosis uncertainty.
- Severe COPD.
- Onset of cor pulmonale.
- Assessment for O_2 therapy, long-term nebuliser or oral steroid therapies.
- Rapid decline in FEV_1.
- Assessment for pulmonary rehab.
- Bullous lung disease.
- Assessment for surgical options – lung transplantation, lung volume reduction surgery.
- Dysfunctional breathing.
- < 40 years old or family history of α-1-antitrypsin deficiency.
- Symptoms disproportionate to lung function deficit.
- Haemoptysis – exclude bronchial cancer.
- Frequent infections – exclude bronchiectasis.

Consultation Models

1987 R. Neighbour: 'The Inner Consultation'

Roger Neighbour's five checklist stages are:

1. **Connecting** – establishing rapport with the patient. This refers to rapport building and may include skills such as acceptance set, curtain raiser/opening gambit, internal search, matching, NLP and speech censoring.

2. **Summarising** – getting to the point of why the patient has come, using skills of eliciting to discover their (ICE) ideas, concerns and expectations and summarising back to the patient. The listening and eliciting skills include the patient is right to start with, explain why you are asking, be facilitative and encouraging (with open-ended questions, statements, my friend), John, echoing and checking.

3. **Handing over** – doctor's and patient's agenda agreed. Skills include negotiating, influencing (doctor's apostolic function) and gift-wrapping ('you don't need those nasty antibiotics this time').

4. **Safety-netting** – 'What if?' predicting skills – what would the doctor do in each case.

5. **Housekeeping** – Taking care of yourself – Am I in good enough shape for the next patient? Get up and stretch, have a cup of coffee, go to the loo.

1984 D. Pendleton: 'The Consultation, An Approach to Learning and Teaching'

The seven tasks to an ideal consultation are:

1. To define the reason for the patient's attendance, including:

    a. the nature and history of the problems

    b. their cause

    c. the patient's ideas, concerns and expectations

    d. the effects of the problems.

2. To consider other problems:

    a. at-risk factors

    b. continuing problems

3. To choose with the patient an appropriate action for each problem.

4. To achieve a shared understanding of the problem with the patient.

5. To involve the patient in the management plan and encourage the patient to accept appropriate responsibility.

6. To use time and resources appropriately:

a. in the consultation

b. in the long term

7. To establish or maintain a relationship with the patient which helps to achieve the other tasks.

1981 C. Helman's Folk Model

Cecil Helman is a medical anthropologist and suggests that a patient with a problem comes to a doctor seeking answers to six questions:

1. What has happened?

2. Why has this happened?

3. Why to me?

4. Why now?

5. What would happen if nothing was done about it?

6. What should I do about it or whom should I consult for further help?

1979 Stott and Davis

A	B
Management of presenting problems	Modification of help-seeking behaviours
C	D
Management of continuing problems	Opportunistic health promotion

1976 Byrne and Long: 'Doctors Talking to Patients'

A study of 2500 audio-taped consultations led to a description of six phases that occur in a consultation:

1. The doctor establishes a relationship with the patient.

2. The doctor either attempts to discover or actually discovers the reason for the patient's attendance.

3. The doctor conducts a verbal or physical examination or both.

4. The doctor, or the doctor and the patient, or the patient considers the condition.

5. The doctor and occasionally the patient details treatment or further investigation.

6. The consultation is terminated usually by the doctor.

1975 J. Heron: 'Six Category Intervention Analysis'

Heron is a humanist psychologist who described the behaviour of health professionals or the interventions of a doctor as one of six interventions:

1. Prescriptive – giving advice or instructions, being critical or directive.
2. Information – imparting new knowledge, instructing or interpreting.
3. Confrontational – challenging a restrictive attitude or behaviour, giving direct feedback within a caring context
4. Cathartic – seeking to release emotion in the form of weeping, laughter, trembling or anger.
5. Catalytic – encouraging the patient to discover and explore his/her own latent thoughts and feelings.
6. Supportive – offering comfort and approval, affirming the patient's intrinsic value.

1966 E. Berne: 'Games People Play'

1. Transactional Analysis – he classifies the states of mind as parent, adult and child and that an individual has a given repertoire of behaviour corresponding to this state of mind.
2. The Child – spontaneous or dependent. Many GP consultations are conducted between a parental doctor and a child-like patient and may not be in the best interests of the patient. The doctor should be aware of transactional analysis and be flexible enough to change his repertoire to avoid consultations degenerating into the games people play.
3. The Adult – this logical ego state is concerned with problem solving, taking in data and processing, and storing knowledge and skills.
4. The Parent – critical or caring, nurturing or controlling.

The transactions during consultations may be complementary, crossed or ulterior.

1957 M. Balint: 'The Doctor, His Patient and The Illness'

The three main themes are: (i) psychological problems are often manifested physically and physical disease causes psychological problems; (ii) doctors have feelings too and these feelings can impact on the consultation process, and (iii) doctors can be trained in a limited way to be more sensitive to what is going on in the patient's mind.

Balintian concepts:

1. The doctor as a drug.

2. The child as the presenting complaint – ticket of entry.

3. Elimination by appropriate physical examination.

4. Collusion of anonymity – nobody taking final responsibility for the patient.

5. The flash – the real reason for attendance is made apparent to both the doctor and the patient.

6. The mutual investment company – the patient presents with episodic offers of both physical and psychological problems in a long relationship.

Contraception

Guidelines for missed pills by > 12 hours

Pill number in pack	Pill(s) missed	Recommended action
1–7	Missed 1 pill	Take the last missed pill Use condoms for 7 days
	Missed 2 or more pills in any combination + UPSI	Take last missed pill but leave other missed pills in the pack. Take further pills as usual. Consider emergency contraception if UPSI after third day in such prolonged pill-free interval + condoms for 7 days
8–14	Missed up to 3 pills + UPSI	Take last missed pill but leave other missed pills in the pack. Take further pills as usual. Use condoms for 7 days. No emergency contraception
	Missed 4 or more pills + UPSI	Emergency contraception may be required + condoms for 7 days
15–21	Missed any one or more of these pills	Start next packet immediately with no break + condoms for 7 days If not seen until after pill-free interval following missed pills, consider emergency contraception

If there are seven or more pills left in the pack after the missed and delayed pills, leave the usual 7-day pill-free break before starting the new pack.

If there are less than seven pills left in the pack after the missed and delayed pills, start the new pack the next day and omit the pill-free break (inactive pills if you have a 28-day pack).

Emergency contraception

< 72 hours after UPSI   Levonelle-2 (levonorgestrel) one tablet now and one in 12 hours

3–5 days after UPSI   Copper IUCD up to day 15 of a lengthened pill-free interval

Critical Reading Protocol (Mnemonic – IMROD)

Introduction (TBOAR)

A. **T**itle, author, institution (English, foreign), journal (respectable, peer-reviewed).

B. **B**ackground (to study).

C. **O**riginality (idea behind the study).

D. **A**ims (clearly stated). Does the study match up to the aims?

E. **R**elevance (to general practice).

Methods (DOS)

A. **D**esign (longitudinal/cross-sectional, observational/experimental, qualitative/quantitative, retrospective/prospective).

    i. Is the study design appropriate? Repeatable?

    ii. Are the instruments and questionnaires reliable (same result if repeated) and validated (answers the research question)?

    iii. Are the confounding variables dealt with?

    iv. Is there a gold standard for comparison?

B. **O**utcome measures (criteria appropriate/clearly defined?)

    i. Are the end-points soft or hard and appropriate?

    ii. Are all the relevant outcomes included?

    iii. Is it truly blind to clinicians and patients?

C. **S**ubjects (inclusion and exclusion criteria clear?)

    i. Is it representative of the population in question? Are they similar in age, sex, ethnic distribution and socioeconomic class?

    ii. Was there use of controls? Was the use of controls appropriate?

    iii. Was the selection of subjects and controls without bias?

    iv. Is the sample size sufficient to detect significant statistical results?

    v. Has the power been calculated?

    vi. Has the sample been unchanged?

    vii. Does the method of randomisation allow reproduction of the experiment?

    viii. Is the treatment plan clear?

    ix. Has the time-span been defined and is it appropriate?

Results (TURDS)

A. **T**ables and graphs.
   Understandable and clear. Is the data represented accurately?

B. **R**esponse rate reasonable > 70%?

C. **D**ropouts – Have the characteristics of the dropouts (failure to respond, non-attenders) been defined? Are all the subjects accounted for?

D. **S**tatistics – has the statistical analysis used been clear and appropriate for the design of the study? Do they include confidence limits and is the P value < 0.05?

Discussion (CACA)

A. **C**ritical evaluation of results – Have the results been discussed with respect to other literature or compared to prior research? Have the applicability and limitations been discussed?

B. **A**ims – met?

C. **C**onclusions – consistent with results, justified with realistic speculations?

D. **A**pplicability – to your population. Is it likely to change your practice?

Others (CORE)

A. **C**onflicts of interest – acknowledged source of funding (pharmaceutical)?

B. **O**verall – clear, ethical, valid, worthwhile study. Are conclusions affordable, available and sensible for your practice?

C. **R**eferences – current?

D. **E**thics – local ethical committee approval?

Depression
Edinburgh Postnatal Depression Questionnaire

This topic is a favourite MCQ module question.

Underline the answer which comes closest to how you have felt in the past 7 days:

1. I have been able to laugh and see the funny side of things:

    As much as I always could.

    Not quite as much.

    Definitely not as much.

    Not at all.

2. I have looked forward with enjoyment to things:

    As much as I ever did.

    Rather less than I used to.

    Definitely less than I used to.

    Hardly at all.

3. I have blamed myself unnecessarily when things went wrong:

    Yes, most of the time.

    Yes, some of the time.

    Not very often.

    No, never.

4. I have been anxious or worried for no good reason:

    No, not at all.

    Hardly ever.

    Yes, sometimes.

    Yes, very often.

5. I have felt scared or panicky for no good reason:

    Yes, quite a lot.

    Yes, sometimes.

    No, not much.

    No, not at all.

6. Things have been getting on top of me:

   Yes, most of the time I have not been able to cope at all.

   Yes, sometimes I have not been coping as well as usual.

   No, most of the time I have coped quite well.

   No, I have been coping as well as ever.

7. I have been so unhappy that I have had difficulty sleeping:

   Yes, most of the time.

   Yes, sometimes.

   Not very often.

   No, not at all.

8. I have felt sad or miserable:

   Yes, most of the time.

   Yes, quite often.

   Not very often.

   No, not at all.

9. I have been so unhappy that I have been crying:

   Yes, most of the time.

   Yes, quite often.

   Only occasionally.

   No, never.

10. The thought of harming myself has occurred to me:

    Yes, quite often.

    Sometimes.

    Hardly ever.

    Never.

Dermatology

Itchy rashes

Contact dermatitis
Itchy form of eczema.
Hairdressers to dye products.
Women to nickel-containing jewellery.
Children to synthetic clothing (polyester, rayon, acrylic, acetate)

Enterobius
Itchy anus due to threadworms. Common in children. Treat with oral mebendazole. May need to repeat treatment in 2 weeks when the eggs hatch.

Lichen planus
Itchy, shiny, violaceous papules with overlying linear white streaks. Koebner phenomenon. Seen in molluscum contagiosum, plane warts, psoriasis and vitiligo.

***Pediculus humanus capitis* (head lice)**
Apply topical aqueous cabaryl 1% liquid or 0.5% lotion, malathion 0.5% liquid or lotion or permethrin 1% cream rinse for 12 hours or overnight and again after 7 days to prevent lice emerging from any surviving eggs.

Sarcoptes scabiei
Intractable pruritus at night to waste products of mites as they burrow in skin. Burrows seen in fingerwebs, flexor aspect of wrists and papules on buttocks and genitalia. Treat all members of household at the same time. Treat with aqueous malathion 0.5% liquid (24 hours) or permethrin 5% dermal cream (8–12 hours) and repeat 1 week later. Do not have a hot bath prior to application of treatment. For infants, young children, elderly and immunocompromised apply also to areas above the neck – scalp, face and ears. Ivermectin is available on a named patient basis for the treatment of Norwegian scabies that is resistant to topical treatment. Itching may persist for up to 6 weeks after treatment.

Tinea (fungal)
Unilateral scaling and fissuring of one palm, feet, groin, body.
Terbinafine is fungicidal vs clotrimazole which is fungistatic.
Tinea capitis (trichophyton) requires oral treatment with griseofulvin, terbinafine or itraconazole syrup for 1 week.

Actinic keratosis (Celtic skin)

- Sunburn to forehead.
- Ablative therapy with Solaraze (topical diclofenac sodium), Efudix bd (fluorouracil) for 6 weeks or cryotherapy (reoccurs as DNA remembers).
- Photodynamic therapy (PDT).

Bullous pemphigoid (elderly)

- Autoimmune watery blisters.
- Diagnosis made on biopsy.
- Treat with prednisolone and azathioprine.
- Versus pemphigus which is very rare.

Bowen's disease (SCC in situ)

- Solitary, painless, flat, occasionally itchy plaque on the lateral lower leg.
- Treat with excision and graft or topical Efudix.

Dermatosis papulosa nigra (DPN)

- Small seborrhoeic warts found on the cheeks and neckline of Africans.
- Refer to dermatology for removal with cautery device.

Eczema (types)

- **Atopic** – flexural and face. Treat with emollients, topical steroids +/− antibiotics for secondary infection. Advise parents to avoid man–made fibres in children's clothing and to buy natural fibres such as cotton, linen, silk and wool. This also applies to bedding. Avoid scented bath additives, soaps, detergents or fabric softeners. New treatment – tacrolimus ointment (protopic) does not cause skin atrophy.
- **Contact** – localised or unilateral. Occupational? Short course of steroids. Refer for patch tests.
- **Discoid** – circular lesions, especially on lower limbs, itchy, may weep with crusting. Treat with potent topical steroid +/− antibiotics. Stress may be trigger.
- **Irritant hand eczema** – finger webs and palms. Water damage. Treat with regular emollients and short periods of topical steroids.
- **Seborrhoeic** – red, scaly plaques on hairline, scalp, eyebrows, sides of nose and anterior chest. Treat with topical antifungal or 1% hydrocortisone, Nizoral or Capasal shampoo.
- **Varicose** – treat underlying venous disease with surgery or compression bandages (after Doppler US has excluded arterial disease). Try emollients and mild topical steroids.

Granuloma annulare

- Flat, smooth purple ring on back of hands, elbows and feet.
- Spontaneous resolution or treat with PUVA to decrease inflammation and mask pigment.

Keloids

- Dressings: Mepiform dressing is available on an FP 10 − rehydrates and allows the keloid to soften and flatten. Leave on until it drops off. Takes 2–3 months to see effect. Cost: 10 dressings = £30. Alternative: silicon dressing.
- Inject with intradermal triamcinolone or offer scar revision surgery.

Necrobiosis lipoidica (diabetes)

- Symmetrical on both lateral sides of shins.
- Treat with intradermal triamcinolone every 4 to 6 weeks (3–4 sessions total).
- Does not correlate with glycaemic control.

Psoriasis

- Trigger factors − stress, smoking, alcohol, anti-malarials, β-blockers, lithium.
- Initial management − emollients, vitamin D analogue cream or ointment (Dovonex to the body and Curatoderm to the face and body). May use Alphosyl HC to face.
- Topical steroids should not be used alone, alternate with vitamin D analogue.
- Scalp psoriasis: Alphosyl or T-Gel shampoo, add topical steroid lotion or vitamin D analogue scalp application. If still problematic massage Cocois into scalp and leave overnight followed by vitamin D or steroid scalp lotion to descale.
- Flexoral psoriasis: trimovate cream/ointment daily for up to 3 weeks
- Palms and soles: dermovate or diprosalic (potent topical steroids) for 6 weeks
- Psoriatic athropathy: diclofenac and refer for systemic therapy
- Refer to dermatologist for:
  - failure to improve after 3–6 months
  - narrow band UVB phototherapy for widespread psoriasis
  - systemic therapy.

- Systemic treatment:

  - methotrexate once weekly for psoriatic arthropathy (avoid aspirin and NSAIDs which affect levels and check LFTs)

  - retinoid (vitamin A)

  - ciclosporin (affects kidney and immunosuppression).

Skin cancer

- **BCC** – Most common type, pearly papule which ulcerates and bleeds. Treat with surgery or radiation.

- **SCC** – Exophytic, indurated, hyperkeratotic firm nodule on lips or ears. Metastasises. The elderly, smokers and renal transplant recipients (on IS drugs) are at risk.

- **Melanoma** – Multiple colours, irregularity and increase in size. Stage with sentinel biopsy. Treat with high dose inteferon, surgery or vaccine trials. Worse prognosis with vertical growth phase vs radical growth phase (little metastatic potential).

Diabetes Type 2: Algorithm for Glycaemic Control

HbA1C 6.5–7.5%

↓

Diet, Education, Exercise, Weight Loss

↙ ↘

BMI < 25 — BMI > 25

BMI < 25

Start metformin regardless of BMI now (UKDS) as it is the only one shown to reduce mortality

↙ ↘

Add metformin (if creatinine < 130) — Add glitazone (check LFTs)

↓ ↓

Start insulin — Start insulin

BMI > 25

Start metformin if creatinine < 130 else lactic acidosis! No longer start with sulphonylurea (only works for 2 years)

↙ ↘

BMI < 30 — BMI > 30

↓ ↓

Add sulphonylurea — Add glitazone

↓ ↓

Start insulin Withdraw sulphonyl Review need for metformin — Start insulin Stop glitazone Review need for metformin

Diabetic Oral Hypoglycaemic Drugs

CLASS	DRUG	MODE OF ACTION	SIDE-EFFECTS
Alpha-glucosidase inhibitor	acarbose	Delays absorption of CHO	Flatulence, diarrhoea, jaundice
Biguanide	metformin	↓ Hepatic glc production	Diarrhoea, metallic taste, abdominal pain, lactic acidosis, ↓ vitamin B_{12} absorption
Insulin sensitisers (thiazolidinediones)	pioglitazone (Actos)	↓ Insulin resistance and resensitise body to its own insulin	GI upset, visual disturbance, anaemia
	rosiglitazone (Avandia)		GI upset, anaemia
Postprandial glucose regulators	nateglinide (Starlix) repaglinide	stimulate insulin secretion by β-cells	hypersensitivity, hypoglycaemia
Sulphonylureas	gliclazide (short-acting)	stimulate insulin secretion by β cells	GI disturbance, hypersensitivity, liver function disorder
	glibenclamide		Avoid in elderly
	glimepiride		
	glipizide		
	gliquidone		
	tolbutamide (short-acting)		Headache, tinnitus
	chlorpropamide		Avoid in elderly (↑ risk of hypoglycaemic attack), facial flushing, ↑ ADH secretion, most side-effects ↓ Na

Drug Misuse and Dependence

Guidelines on Clinical Management. Department of Health Orange Book 1999

Prevalence:

- Male to female ratio of 3 : 1.

- Heroin is main drug of misuse in 55% of cases.

- Methadone, cannabis and amphetamines in declining order of misuse.

- Injecting drug misusers are 22 times more likely to die than non-injectors.

Treatment:

- Reduce the risk of HIV, hepatitis B and C and other blood-borne infections from injecting.

- Reduce the need for criminal activity.

- Reduce the use of illicit drugs by the individual.

- Assist the patient to remain healthy and stabilise patient on substitute medication.

- Shared care with GPs, specialist GPs, community psychiatric nurses, clinical psychologists, pharmacist, social workers and drug and alcohol workers.

- Specialist services required for patients with dual diagnoses (mental illness + drug/alcohol), liver disease, chaotic lifestyle, serious forensic history, unresponsive to oral substitute prescriptions, specialised residential rehabilitation programmes.

Assessment:

- Confirm patient is taking drugs (history, examination and urine toxicology screen).

- Assess degree of dependence (smoking, injecting, amount per week).

- Identify complications of drug misuse and assess risk behaviour (skin abscesses, history of DVT).

- Identify medical, social and mental health problems.

- Offer advice on harm minimisation (clean needle exchange centres, testing for HIV and immunisation against hepatitis B).

- Determine the patient's expectations and degree of motivation.

- Assess the appropriate level of expertise needed for this patient (shared care).
- Determine the need for substitute medication such as methadone or Subutex (buprenorphine).
- Notify the patient to the local Regional Drug Misuse Database (form completion).

History and physical examination:

- Presentation – pregnant, impending court case, wanting help, etc.
- Past and current drug use – age at starting, types, quantity, frequency and routes of administration, overdoses, abstinences, symptoms (hallucinations, fits).
- History of injecting, risk of HIV and hepatitis.
- Medical history – abscess, DVT, chest infections, dental disease, TB, bacterial endocarditis, PE, LMP, last smear, accidents.
- Psychiatric history – admissions, OPC, overdoses, depression or concomitant psychosis (delusions or hallucinations), self-harm, attempted suicide.
- Forensic history – probation, criminal record, outstanding charges.
- Social history – family, children, employment, accommodation (hostel), debt.
- Past contact with treatment services – prior attempts at rehabilitation, methadone, etc.
- Others – drug misuse in partner or family.
- Examine sites of injection for infection (neck, arms, groin and legs).

Investigations:

- Hb, creatinine, LFTs, hepatitis B and C, HIV antibody.
- Urine toxicology test (opiates persist for 24 hours and methadone for 48 hours).

Prescribing doctor:

- No more than 1 week's supply should be dispensed at one time.
- Keep clearly written or computer records of prescribing.
- Monitor patient with regular urine toxicology tests to ensure compliance with substitute drugs.
- A multidisciplinary approach to drug treatment is essential.
- Prescribe methadone in opiate dependence and diazepam in benzodiazepine dependence. Lofexidine is useful for the treatment of withdrawal in a supervised community, inpatient or residential setting.

Opiate withdrawal:

- Peaks at 36–72 hours.

- Presents with sweating, lacrymation, rhinorrhoea, yawning, feeling hot and cold, anorexia, abdominal cramps, tremor, nausea, vomiting or diarrhoea, insomnia, aches and pains, dilated pupils, hypertension and tachycardia.

- Detoxification with methadone mixture 1 mg/ml (initial daily dose of 10–40 mg) or Subutex (buprenorphine). An 8 mg tablet of Subutex is equivalent to 30 mg of methadone. Commence at 2 mg od.

Dyspepsia

1. **Age for endoscopy** – for new dyspepsia has been changed from **45 years to 55 years** in line with national cancer referral guidance. NICE guidelines 2004 now does not specify age criteria.

2. **Test and treat** – the new recommendation is to treat patients < 55 years with uncomplicated dyspepsia on the basis of a +*Helicobacter pylori* test and not to 'test and scope'.

3. **^{13}C urea breath tests** – the **best test** for identification and for confirmation of eradication of *H. pylori* is the ^{13}C urea breath test.

4. **Use of proton pump inhibitors** – continue to follow NICE guidance.

Common causes of dyspepsia:

Duodenal ulcer (+*H. pylori*)	10–15%
Gastric ulcer (+*H. pylori*)	5–10%
Oesophago/gastric CA (+*H. pylori*)	2%
Oesophagitis	10–17%
Gastritis, duodenitis (+*H. pylori*) or hiatus hernia	30%
Normal	30%

Testing for HP:

Serology is simple, widely available and has a high sensitivity but is less accurate than the urea breath test. Routine endoscopy for diagnosis of *H. pylori* is not recommended.

Endoscopy:

For new onset of uncomplicated dyspepsia if > 55 years (withhold anti-secretory drugs for 4 weeks before scope) and for patients with alarm symptoms if < 55 years.

Endoscopy is inappropriate for: duodenal ulcer, which has responded symptomatically to treatment; patients < 55 years; patients who have recently undergone satisfactory endoscopy for same symptoms.

Alarm symptoms:

- Dysphagia and odynophagia.
- Epigastric mass.
- GI bleed.

- Persistent continuous vomiting.

- Prior gastric surgery.

- Prior gastric ulcer.

- Suspicious barium meal.

- Unexplained iron deficiency anaemia.

- Unintentional weight loss ($\geq$ 3 kg).

Treatment for HP:

- **Duodenal ulcer +HP** – 1 week triple tx with PPI (bd) or RBC (ranitidine bismuth citrate) + amoxicillin 500 mg –1 g bd or metronidazole 400–500 mg bd + clarithromycin 500 mg bd; quadruple tx for second-line tx with PPI + bismuth 120 mg qds + metronidazole 400–500 mg tds + tetracycline 500 mg qds

- **Duodenal ulcer no HP** – cimetidine 800 mg nocte; refer GI if not NSAID-ulcer.

- **Gastric ulcer + HP** – HeliClear (lansoprazole) + antisecretory tx for 2 months. NICE advises COX2 specific antagonists if need NSAIDs. Long-term PPI or misoprostol if on NSAIDs.

- **Gastric ulcer no HP** – antisecretory tx for 2/12. Stop NSAIDs. Give PPI if on NSAID.

- **Oesophagitis** – 4 weeks of antacids, raft preparations (alginate), H_2R antagonists, or prokinetic agents (cisapride).

- Response to PPI and H_2R antagonists is better if dyspepsia is ulcer-like or reflux.

ECGs

Be able to recognise these ECG changes for the MCQ module of the MRCGP exam.

Acute pericarditis:

- Diffuse ECG changes in all leads except lead V_1 and aVR.
- Scooping/concave ST segment – convexity is downwards.
- ST elevation.
- Blunted T wave.

Myocardial infarction:

- Anterior MI – Q waves in V_1-V_4.
- Inferior MI – Q waves in leads II, III and aVF.
- Lateral MI – Q waves in I, aVL, V_5, V_6 and V_2.
- ST elevation or depression.
- ST segment is flat, scooped or shows coving (convexity is upwards).
- Local ECG changes.
- Time scale:

– 0 minutes	normal – left-sided leads always have Q waves
– minutes	peak T waves (ischaemia), hyperacute T waves
– minutes–hours	ST elevation with coving (injury)
– minutes–hours	T wave inversion
– hours–days	Q wave (myocardial infarct, necrosis) in an abnormal lead which is ≥ 0.4 seconds wide and contributes quarter too much to QRS
– days–weeks	Q wave remains forever, ST segment returns to normal, T wave inversion reverses

Pulmonary embolism:

- $S_1 Q_3$ pattern.
- Inverted T in leads V_1-V_4.
- ST depression in lead II.
- Transient RBBB, right axis deviation.

ENT
(Everything You Wanted to Know)

Know the anatomy of the tympanic membrane (a particular favourite MCQ)

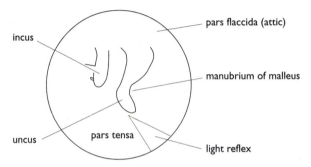

ENT definitions (a favourite matching question)

- **Acoustic neuroma** – tumour of the VIIIth cranial nerve in the internal acoustic meatus. Presents with either unilateral sensorineural hearing loss or tinnitus.

- **Attic cholesteatoma** – overgrowth of squamous epithelial cells from the attic of TM (pars flaccida) into the middle ear via an attic or posterior marginal TM perforation. The potential complication is erosion of bone, involvement of the dura and intracranial spread. Urgent referral. Surgical procedure: mastoidectomy, but limited by waiting list times of up to a year!

- **Aural polyp** – chronic discharging ear. Associated with longstanding TM perforation and chronic suppurative otitis media. Surgical procedure: aural polypectomy and mastoid operation.

- **Bell's palsy** – diagnosis of exclusion; involves the forehead (LMN: VIIth palsy); urgent referral to ENT for PTA hearing test; prescribe eye drops and eye pad nocte; treat with tapering dose of prednisolone – 80 mg, 60 mg, 40 mg, 20 mg, 10 mg od.

- **Erysipelas** – haemolytic streptococci enter through skin fissures or active otitis externa. Treat with IV benzylpenicillin.

- **Facial palsy** – congenital (forceps); metabolic (hyperthyroidism, malignant OE, pregnancy); infection (lyme disease, OE, OM, chickenpox, mastoiditis); neoplasm (cholesteatoma, parotid or basal cell CA, VIIth nerve tumour); toxic (diphtheria, tetanus, thalidomide); trauma (head injury, temporal bone fracture, MVA); iatrogenic (postmastoidectomy, inferior dental block, rabies vaccine); idiopathic and neurological (Bell's palsy, Guillain–Barré, multiple sclerosis).

- **Grommets** – plastic tubes placed through an anterior-inferior TM myringotomy for treatment of glue ear (secretory otitis media). These dislodge spontaneously after 12–18 months.

- **Herpes zoster (Ramsey–Hunt syndrome)** – facial nerve palsy, vesicles in EAM.

- **Malignant otitis externa** – deep otalgia with granulation tissue blocking the EAM; found in diabetics; may affect CN VII–XII and lead to osteomyelitis, brain abscess and death; offending organism is *Pseudomonas pyocaneus* which is investigated with CT scan and granulation tissue biopsy and treated with IV antibiotics.

- **Ménière's disease** – nausea, vertigo, low-frequency sensorineural hearing loss; with each attack, hearing does not recover, may be bilateral.

- **Nasal polyps** – benign grey opalescent 'peeled grapes'; ask about coexistent asthma and aspirin sensitivity; treat with topical steroid nasal sprays/drops; arrange CT scan of sinuses; may need FESS operation.

- **Noise-induced hearing loss** – recruitment, 4 Hz.

- **Osteomas** – swimmer's osteoma, bony hard swellings in the meatus, hyperostosis. Complications include wax build up and otitis externa. Surgical intervention: removal with microdrill.

- **Otitis media** – treat with ibuprofen if < 24 hours with fever and red TM. If > 24 hours, with a temperature greater than 40°C and bulging red TM, treat with amoxicillin. Conductive hearing loss. Beware of postnasal space neoplasm in adults with unilateral secretory otitis media. Adenoidal hypertrophy leads to Eustachian tube dysfunction and otitis media with effusion infections in children.

- **Otosclerosis** – conductive hearing loss with normal TM; commonly presents during pregnancy. Paracusis willisi – hears better in a noisy environment

- **Presbyacusis** – gradual bilateral high-frequency sensorineural hearing loss with age.

- **Secretory otitis media with retraction** – golden or brown eardrum; prominent malleus; watchful waiting; 40 dB conductive hearing loss on PTA with flat tympanometry; surgical intervention: grommets + EUA PNS +/– adenoidectomy.

- **Ramsay–Hunt syndrome** – herpes zoster virus involves the geniculate ganglion of the VIIth cranial nerve; associated with facial palsy and SNHL. Treat with aciclovir 800 mg 5 times a day, analgesia, Pope wick and steroid otic drops.

- **Tympanosclerosis** – incidental finding of a chalk-like or cotton-wool appearance to TM. Check if there is a past history of otitis media. No treatment required.

ENT emergency referrals for admission

1. Acute tonsillitis:

- Not eating or drinking, drooling saliva, +/− trismus.

- Admit, swabs not routinely performed, FBC and Monospot, IVIs, IV benzylpenicillin 1.2 g qds and metronidazole 500 mg tds, analgaesia − IM pethidine and diclofenac, soluble co-codamol.

- Send home on a 1 week course of penicillin 500 mg qds and metronidazole 400 mg tds and dispersible diclofenac and soluble co-codamol.

- **Indications for tonsillectomy** − four or five episodes of tonsillitis a year, time off work/school, two episodes of quinsy a year, unilateral enlargement of tonsil (need to perform tonsillectomy to exclude lymphoma).

- **Complications and readmission post tonsillectomy** − 10% risk of secondary haemorrhage (postoperative bleeding due to infection 7−10 days later) which is treated with antibiotics if the bleeding from the tonsillar fossa is minimal and IV antibiotics if the bleeding is more than a cupful. This rarely needs a second operation to stem the bleeding. Prevention − advise the patient to eat and drink post-operatively (community nurse can give analgaesia in suppository form if child refuses the oral route).

2. Infectious mononucleosis (glandular fever):

- Not eating or drinking, drooling saliva, trismus, flu-like symptoms, muscle fatigue, teenager, contact through kissing.

- White membrane covers one or both tonsils.

- Admit FBC and Monospot looking for heterophile antibodies, IVIs, IV benzylpenicillin 1.2 g qds and metronidazole 500 mg tds, add 8 mg IV dexamethasone, soluble co-codamol or dispersible Voltarol (diclofenac sodium) and IM analgaesia.

- Antibiotics are prescribed to cover superimposed secondary bacterial infection. Do EBV serology (anti-EBNA 1 IgG) in children < 10 years, as < 10% have a positive reaction.

- 90% have a negative Monospot test (false negative rate = 90%) and still have glandular fever. If the patient is a professional athlete, obtain an ultrasound of the spleen before clearing the patient for full contact sports to exclude splenomegaly or spontaneous splenic rupture.

- If confirm positive Monospot, advise the patient to avoid contact sports for 6 weeks and give time off work/school; send home on oral antibiotics for 1 week.

3. Quinsy:

- Unilateral painful and inflamed tonsil with cellulitis or abscess.

- Squirt lidocaine (lignocaine) spray to the back of the throat and aspirate with a 18G needle and syringe. Admit for IVIs, IV benzylpenicillin + metronidazole, and analgaesia.

4. Severe epistaxis:

- Risk factors (hypertension SBP > 160, aspirin, warfarin).

- Anterior bleed (from Little's area on the septum). Treatment plan – cautery with silver nitrate sticks or pressure to nasal vestibule.

- Posterior bleed (serious!). Risk groups: elderly, atherosclerotic vessels, hypertensives. Px – nasal packing with 8 cm Merocel (tampon) or balloons (Brighton or urinary catheter), squirt Otrivene nasal decongestant (xylometazoline hydrochloride) to inflate the Merocel. Admit, resuscitate and transfuse if necessary. Control hypertension with nifedipine SR and give Valium (diazepam) 2–5 mg tds.

Emergency ENT clinic referrals

1. Foreign bodies:

- Ear – if it is a live insect, instil lidocaine (lignocaine) into the ear canal to kill the insect. Refer all cases of FBs in the ear to the emergency ENT clinic for removal under the microscope. If the child is too young to remain still under the microscope, he or she will be placed on the next available elective list for EUA and removal.

- Nose – positioning is key in a child. If the object is in the nasal vestibule, this can be removed. If it is beyond the vestibule, refer the patient to the emergency ENT clinic and the child will be booked on the next available elective list for EUA and removal. If the child has a persistent unilateral nasal discharge and signs of vestibulitis, refer the patient to the emergency ENT clinic as the child may need EUA for suspected FB.

- Throat (fishbone) – usually seen in the tonsil bed, base of tongue, vallecula (between the tongue and epiglottis) or the piriform fossa (on either side of the larynx). The latter two sites require a GA for removal. The fishbone may be seen on soft tissue lateral neck x-ray. Advise the patient to eat bread to dislodge the fishbone. Refer patient to the emergency ENT clinic for flexible nasoendoscopy. If nothing is seen, advise soluble paracetamol and rescope in 3–5 days if still symptomatic. Could be pain from a scratch to the mucosa which heals conservatively.

- Throat (food bolus stuck in the upper oesophagus) – give IM Buscopan (hyoscine butyl bromide) and Valium (diazepam) to relax oesophageal muscle, give fizzy drinks. If no success and the patient is in pain and drooling saliva, or if the bolus contains bone, arrange x-ray, admit for rigid oesophagoscopy on the emergency list. If it is in the lower oesophagus, the general surgeons can perform flexible oesophagoscopy.

- Throat (50 pence coin stuck in the cricopharyngeal sphincter) – confirm on x-ray, admit and list for emergency EUA and removal with rigid oesophagoscopy.

2. Otitis externa:

- Refer when the patient has profuse otorrhoea requiring microsuction or if the external auditory meatus is swollen preventing adequate instillaton of ear drops.

- Microsuction +/− insertion of Pope wick with Sofradex (dexamethasone) 4 drops tds for 10 days. Use cotton wool to prevent leakage of drops. In adults and children, in particular, Otomize (dexamethasone) spray is an alternative and a personal favourite and comes with a custom ear nozzle for ease of application. Other choices for otitis externa include Otosporin (hydrocortisone) and Gentisone HC (hydrocortisone). For suspected *Pseudomonas aeruginosa* infection (dirty water) and distinctive malodorous discharge add ciprofloxacin but advise patient of potential photosensitivity rash.

- Prevention – advise patients not to use cotton buds (as ears are self-cleaning), not to swim, and not to get ears wet (use Vaseline (petroleum jelly) on cotton wool) during treatment.

- Beware malignant otitis externa in a diabetic (granulation tissue occluding the external auditory canal) which presents with deep otalgia or associated VII–XIIth cranial nerve palsies.

3. Acute otitis media:

- Refer the patient for admission if concerned the patient may have acute mastoiditis (complication of untreated otitis media – rare with advent of antibiotics). The pinna will be positioned forward and downwards in comparison to the good ear.

4. Perforated tympanic membrane:

- The patient will complain of a whistling sound in the ear. Advise the patient to keep the ear dry, give augmentin or amoxicillin for 1 week and refer to the next available emergency ENT clinic.

- In ENT clinic, the perforation will be confirmed by inspection. Small perforations heal within 6 weeks. The patient will be brought back to a routine outpatient clinic for a pure tone audiogram, which should show resolution of a conductive hearing loss and healing perforation. If the perforaton is total or subtotal, and the patient's lifestyle is compromised (swimmer or airline pilot), a tympanoplasty is offered.

- Note – ENT doctors do prescribe antibiotic eardrops, i.e. Sofradex (dexamethasone) for patients with TM perforations. However, avoid

Gentisone HC (hydrocortisone) antibiotic eardrops, sodium bicarbonate drops and diluted H_2OH for wax build up in patients with TM perforations as the drops will burn.

5. Sudden onset unilateral sensorineural hearing loss:

- This is often of unknown aetiology but may be due to exposure to, for example, the mumps virus if the person is a schoolteacher. Need to exclude acoustic neuroma (tumour of the CPA VIIIth nerve).

- Pure tone audiogram and tympanometry are performed to confirm unilateral sensorineural hearing loss. If the onset is acute, i.e. within the past 24 hours, the patient is admitted for hourly carbonox treatment (5% CO_2 and 95% O_2) and given oral betahistine, a vasodilator. An MRI scan is arranged to exclude acoustic neuroma.

6. Bell's palsy:

- Lower motor neurone facial palsy of unknown aetiology (55%). Diagnosis of exclusion – need to exclude herpes zoster oticus (Ramsay–Hunt syndrome), trauma, tumour of the parotid gland or facial nerve schwannoma, otitis media, multiple sclerosis, sarcoid, drugs, etc.

- Perform a full neurological examination. Inspect the ears for vesicles to exclude Ramsay–Hunt syndrome. Arrange pure tone audiogram and tympanogram. Give high-dose steroids tapered over 1 week if acute onset, i.e. prednisolone 60 mg od 2 days, 40 mg od 2 days, 20 mg od 2 days, 10 mg od 2 days. Eye patch to be worn at night and eye ointment. Elderly have a poorer prognosis for recovery.

7. Subperichondrial haematoma:

- Usually as a result of blunt trauma to the ear while boxing or playing rugby.

- This will need to be aspirated and a pressure dressing applied to avoid cauliflower ear from degeneration of the cartilage.

8. Broken nose:

- X-ray is not mandatory. Diagnosis is made on palpation. The patient is seen at least 5 days after the event to properly assess once the swelling has abated. The patient can then be listed for MUA on an elective list. The caveat is that this must be performed within 12 days of the injury. If the patient also has a deviated nasal septum or one that has dislocated off the maxillary crest, the patient will have to wait 6 months for septorhinoplasty or septoplasty.

- Complication of blunt trauma to nose – septal haematoma is blood under the subperichondrium. The patient complains of bilateral blocked nose (total nose obstruction), and on examination there are bilateral cherry red swellings in the nose. These are extremely tender to palpate. This will need urgent EUA and I+D to prevent septal cartilage necrosis. Partial obstruction does not require treatment. The complication of untreated septal haematoma is saddle nose.

ENT 'pearls of wisdom'

- **Beware** of persistent unilateral conductive hearing loss and nasal blockage in the adult – need to exclude tumour of the nasopharynx.

- **Beware** of cheek swelling in the absence of tooth root infection – maxillary cancer.

- **Beware** of an attic retraction pocket in the pars flaccida region of the eardrum; if a dry crust is present, this will need gentle removal under the microscope to inspect for cholesteatoma (skin in the middle ear cleft).

- **Beware** of hoarseness persisting more than 6 weeks. I have seen a case of laryngeal CA in a non-smoker in her twenties.

- **Beware** of 'cotton-wool' sitting on the eardrum. This could just be incidental tympanosclerosis.

ENT outpatient clinic referrals

Ears

1. Glue ear (otitis media with effusion):

- Conservative management includes Otovent device (bought at the chemist), Rynacrom (sodium cromoglicate), etc.

- Indications for grommets include 3 months of conductive hearing loss $\geq$ 40 dB, interference with school or recurrent ear infections. Potential risks are repeat grommet insertion and permanent tympanic membrane perforation.

2. Otosclerosis:

- Conductive hearing loss associated with a normal TM. Familial. Often presents in pregnancy. Hearing is improved in noisy environments. Perform pure tone audiometry and tympanometry. May be associated with blue sclerae.

- Surgical procedure – stapedectomy (stapedius implant).

3. Vertigo (cardiac, positional/musculoskeletal or hearing disorder):

- Enquire if history of cardiovascular disease? History of neck or back pain, hearing loss or tinnitus? Unsteady vs room spinning? Reaching for an item on the top shelf elicits vertigo? In/out of bed (positional). Perform neurological examination, Romberg's and Unterberger's (marching in place with eyes shut and arms extended) tests, pure tone audiometry and tympanometry, caloric testing.

- Differential diagnosis: benign positional vertigo (Hallpike's manouevre); Meniere's disease (hearing loss, vertigo and tinnitus) with each attack causing worsening of baseline hearing and lasts minutes to hours; acute vestibular failure lasts hours to days and precedes an URTI; multiple sclerosis; aminoglycosides, metronidazole; acoustic neuroma; cholesteatoma; vertebrobasilar insufficiency.

- Treatment includes vestibular rehabilitation with an auditory physiotherapist (Cooksey–Cawthorne exercises to retrain the inner ear); medical treatment with vestibular sedatives (Stemetil (prochlorperazine), cinnarizine, betahistine or antidepressants). Try to wean patient off dependency on vestibular sedatives.

- Tinnitus arises anywhere from the brainstem to the auditory cortex (not solely from the ear). *Gingko biloba* herbal remedy is no better than a placebo. Tinnitus retraining therapy may be offered. I suggest patients use ocean sounds in the bedroom to block the tinnitus. Unilateral tinnitus must be investigated with MRI to exclude acoustic neuroma.

4. Dewaxing:

- Treat wax build up with sodium bicarbonate drops for 2 weeks or use diluted hydrogen peroxide. Ear syringing at GP practice, however this puts patient at risk of otitis externa. Advise patients not to use cotton buds, as this will lead to increased hard, brown-black wax. ENT OPC can offer microsuction of wax, however this is more appropriate for patients with mastoid cavities who have lost the natural ability of the EAC to remove wax by migration and thus require routine dewaxing.

Nose

1. Nasal polyps:

- Conservative management includes betnesol nasal drops or flixonase ampoules for 6 weeks; prednisolone 5 mg od for 2 weeks or steroid nasal drops (Beconase (beclomethasone dipropionate), Nasacort (triamcinolone acetonide), Nasonex (mometasore furoate). Skin prick allergy testing is performed by the outpatient ENT nurse. Be aware of the triad – aspirin sensitivity, nasal polyps and asthma. Cystic fibrosis is also associated with nasal polyps. Antrochoanal polyp arises within the maxillary antrum and protrudes into the nasopharynx.

- Indications for nasal polypectomy or FESS – failed medical treatment. A CT scan of the sinuses is obtained as the polyps arise from the ethmoid sinuses and can be associated with distortion of the nasal bridge and gross opacity of the maxillary and ethmoid sinuses. In this case a snare polypectomy is not adequate and the patient will require FESS/polypectomy. Warn the patient of risk of injury to the orbit or brain.

2. Rhinitis (allergic):

- Refer for skin prick allergy testing.

- Prescribe Betnesol (betamethasone) 2 drops for 2 weeks, then give Beconase (beclomethasone dipropionate) spray (2 squirts bd) for months. Other sprays include my favourite, Nasacort (triamcinolone acetonide; odourless, thixotropic – sticks to nasal mucosa, once a day with low steroid content and effective within 16 hours, licensed for patients age 6 and above) and Nasonex (mometasone furoate). Rhinolast spray (azelastine hydrochloride, antihistamine nasal spray) for children age 2–12. Sodium cromoglicate (Rynacrom) good in children. Beware Flixonase (fluticasone propionate, highest steroid content for efficacy).

- Prescribe antihistamines after topical treatment has failed.

3. Rhinitis (non-allergic; non-eosinophilic vasomotor):

- Drugs, hormonal, hypothyroidism, menopause, pregnancy, occupational and environmental irritants.

- Prescribe sympathomimetic drugs (pseudoephedrine), topical nasal ipratropium spray (Rinatec) for senile watery rhinorrhoea.

- Surgical option – reduction of inferior turbinates with diathermy.

4. Snoring:

- Assess BMI, advise weight reduction if BMI > 30, reduce alcohol intake, avoid heavy meals at night.

- If due to a deviated nasal septum, offer septoplasty.

- If due to a redundant uvula, offer uvuloplasty.

- If due to a redundant uvula and low hanging posterior pharynx, offer UVPPP.

- Surgical risks include pain, dry throat, voice change, etc.

- Otherwise arrange a sleep study to assess for apnoeic episodes if the BMI is not high.

- Patients with sleep apnoea must be advised not to drive.

- Children who have associated sleep apnoea may benefit from EUA and adenoidectomy. Some advocate concurrent tonsillectomy for obstructive airway.

- Beware of the child with a bifid uvula! That child is most likely to have a submucous cleft, which can be palpated. If adenoidectomy is inadvertently performed in such a child, the child is at high risk of rhinolalia aperta (Mickey Mouse voice). If the child has singing aspirations, warn that adenoidectomy may change the quality of the voice. I advise parents that most children under the age of 6 snore, as the size of the adenoids and tonsils are large in comparison to the size of the skull and that snoring disappears as the size of the head grows and the adenoids shrink in comparison. I have found that children who have had tonsillectomy are more prone to catching viral infections.

5. Acute and chronic sinusitis:

- Manage with antibiotics (between 2 and 6 weeks) and nasal decongestants (Otrivine (xylometazoline)).

- Periorbital cellulitis requires urgent admission, IV antibiotics, urgent ophthalmologist review with visual acuity and colour vision check, and CT scan to exclude optic nerve compression. The patient may need urgent orbital decompression/FESS with diminished visual acuity and affected colour vision.

Throat

1. Recurrent tonsillitis/quinsy

2. Hoarseness:

- In children is often associated with voice abuse. EUA of larynx excludes other pathology such as papillomatosis.

- Screamer's nodules can be seen on FNE in adults with voice abuse.

3. Head and neck pathology:

- A slowly growing parotid swelling is most likely benign versus a fast growing parotid swelling associated with facial nerve palsy.

- Alcohol and tobacco are risk factors for head and neck CA.

- Maxillary CA may present with eye, teeth, facial or nasal symptoms which include diplopia, ophthalmoplegia, facial pain, numbness, nasal obstruction, loss of smell, taste, toothache, loose teeth, oroantral fistula, etc.

4. Vocal cord checks:

- Advised for patients undergoing thyroidectomy to ensure the recurrent laryngeal nerve is intact preoperatively.

Eyes (Everything You Wanted to Know)

Age-related macular degeneration

Degeneration of the macular region of the retina leading to loss of central vision.

Dry type (80–95% of cases):

- Non-exudative, painless, slow onset.
- Loss of central vision over months or years.
- Drusen deposits and atrophy of retinal pigment epithelium.
- No available treatment.

Wet type (10% of cases and 90% of sight loss in the UK):

- Exudative.
- Painless, rapid onset with progression of central vision loss.
- Straight lines appear to bend.
- +/− abnormal colour vision.
- Subretinal neovascularisation with haemorrhage and scarring.
- PDT or argon laser only prevents further deterioration.

Cataracts

- Lens opacity. See black shadow on lens at +10 dioptre.
- Babies should be screened for cataracts.
- Exclude metabolic disorder in children with cataracts.
- Implication of surgery for the patient is that the plastic lens cannot focus. So indication for surgery is if cataract prevents patient from doing what they want to do.
- Post-cataract complications – acute ↓ in vision, with pain and red eye is endophthalmitis until proven otherwise. Poor red reflex. Refer promptly.

Chemical injury

- Apply LA and immediate wash out with saline/water 1–2 continuous irrigation for 15–30 minutes.

- Check vision, F-stain = fluorescein stain, pH litmus paper (normal 7.5–8).
- Check cornea to exclude white eye which represents limbal ischaemia (blanched blood vessels) following alkali injury. This can progress to corneal necrosis within 24 hours. Refer urgently.
- If the entire eye stains blue and the eye is white, the patient will need grafts for weeks.
- Cotton bud sweep conjunctiva under lid to wipe off any metal or grit.

Diabetic retinopathy

- Screen pregnant women with diabetes every 4–6 weeks to exclude maculopathy.
- Screen asymptomatic diabetics every 6 months to 1 year.
- **Degree 1: background retinopathy (BDR)** – microaneurysms, no treatment, annual review.
- **Degree 2: preproliferative retinopathy** – cotton wool spots marker for ischaemia, i.e. soft exudates at risk of developing new vessels.
  - **Maculopathy** gives rise to: (i) yellow hard exudates (lipoprotein) – treat with laser same day as seen in eye clinic; (ii) macula oedema – leakage of fluid, treat with laser to decrease visual loss by 50%; (iii) ischaemic (no blood supply) – no treatment.
- **Degree 3: proliferative retinopathy** – new vessels can bleed and result in vitreous haemorrhage or become scar tissue causing traction on the retina and resultant visual loss. Panretinal photocoagulation is used to treat neovascularisation.

Examination

- Visual acuity: near/far, pinhole, +/– glasses.
- Colour vision: Ishihara (lost in optic neuritis, nerve transection or macular degeneration), red desaturation first (red colour is less bright).
- RAPD – relative afferent pupillary defect. Swing light across pupils. If the opposite pupil dilates paradoxically instead of consensual constriction to light, APD is present and indicates injury to the optic nerve. Present in optic neuritis.
- Do not dilate patients with angle closure glaucoma as can precipitate visual loss by sending the elderly patient with a small anterior chamber into angle closure.

Floaters

- If gradually increasing think vitreous degeneration, lens opacity, corneal scar.
- If sudden onset with flashing +/- decrease in vision, think vitreous detachment, embolus in disc, blocked blood vessel or retinal detachment.
- 2 weeks after cataract operation with counting fingers may represent infection, vitreous detachment or haemorrhage, or retinal detachment (dilated fundus examination to exclude). Check for RAPD.

Fundoscopy tips

- Stand 20 cm away to check for red reflex, cataract (lens opacity) or blood in the eye (black reflex–vitreous haemorrhage).
- Look for the optic nerve nasally.
- Look for laser burns inferiorly.
- To see beyond the cataract, dial to −8 (red).
- Use the green beam (red-free light) to check for haemorrhages or microaneurysms, which will appear black.
- Ask the patient to look directly into your light to assess the patient's macula.

Glaucoma

- Asymptomatic until visual fields are impaired.
- Associated with IOP > 21, optic disc cupping and visual field defects.
- For repeat prescriptions for timolol ask the patient if he is having SOB or eye soreness. If he is having beta-blocker side-effects, give Xalatan nocte instead.

Lids

- **Dacrocystitis** – treat with broad-spectrum antibiotics for pus in lacrimal sac. May need dacrocystorhinostomy.
- **Ectropion** – routine referral for minor operation.
- **Entropion** – invert the lid; if corneal transparency is gone, this is an ominous sign and the patient will need to be operated on within a week.
- **Herpes zoster ophthalmicus** – rarely crosses the midline. May see scabs around the eye. If the nose is spared, then the eye is spared.

Treat with acyclovir, but if not, refer urgently as may develop oculomotor palsy and iritis.

- **Meibomian cyst** – the size of a marble; may be removed under LA in OPC.
- **Thyroid disease** – overaction of Muller's muscle with uniocular proptosis.

Orbital injury

- Check VA through a pinhole. Reduced VA may indicate presence of hyphaema or retinal oedema.
- Check optic nerve by checking VA and colour vision.
- If patient has diplopia on looking up and down, consider orbital blowout fracture. Palpate rim for notch of fracture.
- Fixed and dilated pupil indicates increased IOP.
- Small pupil suggests iritis.
- Check EOMI.
- Check for hyphaema and exclude retinal detachment or vitreous haemorrhage.
- Cover test.
- Check for sensation with cotton ball under the eye (infraorbital nerve).
- Check for proptosis, enophthalmos.
- Advise patient not to blow nose as this may cause orbital inflation.
- Check IOP.

Palsy

- In long-sightedness, a convergent squint occurs when not wearing glasses.
- **Lateral rectus palsy (CN VI)** – consider brain tumour, stroke. Limited lateral deviation of eye. May see convergent squint.
- **Sudden onset of painful diplopia, CN III palsy** – cannot look up and out or down and in, eye down and out with lid palsy and dilated pupil, consider compressive lesion, i.e. posterior communicating artery aneurysm or subarachnoid haemorrhage and refer urgently for MRI. Diabetes does not affect the pupil.
- **Sudden onset of CN III palsy in a child** with ptosis and a lateral diverging eye, consider posterior communicating aneurysm.
- **Superior oblique (CN VI) palsy** – eye keeps going down and out on accommodation.

- Bilateral horizontal nystagmus – consider multiple sclerosis.
- Squint in children – do cover test. Use torch and alternate. This will bring out the squint. Orthoptic referral to avoid amblyopia (useless vision).

Pingecula

- Yellow fatty deposit on eye.
- Refer for cosmetic removal.

Pterygion

- Broad-based at 3 or 9 o'clock.
- Takes 50–80 years for pterygia to cover iris.
- Routine referral for removal and conjunctival graft.

Red eye

Conjunctivitis:

- Allergic (itchy and watering) – sodium cromoglicate (Opticrom) eye drops.
- Bacterial – irritation with sticky discharge. Check for preauricular lymph nodes. Treat with chloramphenicol or Fucithalmic (fusidic acid) drops.
- Chlamydial (non-resolving conjunctivitis – consider testing).
- Viral – most common and resolves in 1–2 weeks; adenovirus (pharyngoconjunctival – fever with photophobia, self-limiting, resolves in 2–6 weeks, mandatory 2 weeks off work as highly contagious).
- Check vision and ideally do fluorescein stain of cornea.
- Pupils equal and central, no photophobia, normal VA.

Corneal abrasion/ulcer:

- Contact lens wearer at risk – refer if patient has red eye.
- Do not apply local anaesthetic to a patient with a corneal abrasion, as the patient may rub the eye and make the abrasion larger.
- Recurrent abrasions common in young mothers from finger poking, postmenopausal women and in morning after alcohol binge (dehydration). Treat with lubricants (hypromellose) for 2 months.
- Use fluorescein dye to stain corneal break 'green' and use a blue light to pick up 'dendritic HSV ulcers – green Xmas tree'. Do not use steroid drops in eyes as this proliferates the HSV and prevents graft uptake if needed.

Episcleritis:

- Tender, localised to one segment of the eye. Treat with oral NSAIDs.

Scleritis:

- Severe pain. Requires systemic steroids. Associated with arthritides.

Acute iritis/uveitis:

- Acute red eye, painful (ciliary muscle) with photophobia and an irregular pupil as iris gets stuck. Worsening vision. Ask if the patient has had this before, as the differential includes HLA B27 arthritides, HIV, lyme disease, inflammatory bowel disease, idiopathic, sarcoidosis, toxoplasmosis. Treat with topical steroids and mydriatic drops (cyclopentolate) to rest pupil.

Acute angle closure glaucoma:

- Usually elderly female presents at dusk when pupil dilates and closes off angle. Symptoms include pain, headache, N/V, decreased VA, cloudy cornea, dilated and sluggish/fixed pupil. The eyeball is rock hard on palpation, the pupil fixed, the conjunctiva injected and the vision diminished. Normal IOP is between 10 and 21. You may see a sudden increase of IOP from 20 to 60, as aqueous humour cannot get in front of the iris and so gets occluded behind the iris. The iris then adheres to the back of the cornea. The optic nerve can be damaged within 6 hours. Refer urgently to specialist. Administer antiemetic and IV acetazolamide (Diamox) to decrease aqueous humour production and bring down IOP and release block with pilocarpine drops. Patient has 6–8 hours before vision is lost.

Side-effects of drugs

Beta-blocker	dry eyes
Prednisolone	glaucoma, papilloedema, posterior subcapsular cataract, corneal thinning
Rifampicin	orange-red tears

Sudden painless loss of vision

- Take a history and ask for symptoms of giant cell arteritis, amaurosis fugax, curtain like effect with flashes or floaters (retinal detachment), diabetes +/− laser treatment.
- Check vision, visual fields, RAPD and fundus.

Anterior ischaemic optic neuropathy:

- Elderly.
- Headache.
- Jaw claudication.
- Temporal tenderness.
- Polymyalgia.
- Swollen optic disc on fundoscopy.
- Check ESR and CRP (more sensitive).
- Risk of bilateral visual loss.
- Treat with steroids.

Central retinal artery occlusion:

- History of atrial fibrillation, giant cell arteritis, hypertension.
- Cherry red spot in macula and swollen optic disc.
- No light perception.
- APD.
- Auscultate for carotid bruits.
- Refer immediately for treatment within 6–12 hours to avoid optic nerve atrophy.
- Treat with IV Diamox (acetazolamide), ocular massage, AC paracentesis.

Central retinal vein occlusion:

- Finger counting.
- Large optic disc.
- Stormy sunset with engorged veins.
- Possible improvement to peripheral vision in 6–12 months.
- At risk for new vessel formation.
- No definitive treatment.

Optic neuritis (pain on movement):

- Age 20–45 years.
- Decreased vision and colour vision.
- RAPD.
- +/− disc swelling.
- Unilateral.
- Seen in multiple sclerosis.
- No definitive treatment.

Retinal detachment:

- 3 F's – flashers (flashing lights), floaters (looking through frog spawn) and field defect (half of field).
- Get the patient to lie flat (if cannot see down below and sees flashing lights, suggests upper detachment).
- Urgent referral.

Vitreous haemorrhage:

- Common in diabetics with neovascularisation.
- Seen with retinal detachment and bleeding disorders.
- Spontaneous absorption.
- Treatment: photocoagulation of new vessels.

Fitness To Drive
DVLA Guidelines updated January 2004

Condition	Ordinary car licence Group 1	LGV or PCV Group 2
Age	> 70 years renew with completion of medical questionnaire every 3 years	Medical confirmation of fitness at age 45 and 5-yearly until 65, and then annually
AIDS syndrome	1, 2, 3 year licences with medical review	Maintain CDT count at or > 200 for minimum 6 months. Cases assessed on individual basis
HIV positive	Need not notify DVLA	Need not notify DVLA
Alcohol BAL > 87.5 micrograms/100 ml	Misuse – 6/12 revocation Dependency – 1 year Hepatic cirrhosis – revoke	Off 1 year for misuse Dependency – 3 years Alcohol-related disorder – revoke
Arrhythmia	Cease unless cause controlled for 4/52	Disqualified unless controlled for 3/12 with LVEF > 0.4
Pacemaker implant or angioplasty	1/52 cease	6/52 disqualifies
Angina	Cease until controlled Need not notify	Revocation. Angina-free for 6/52
CABG	Cease for 4/52 Need not notify	Disqualified for 6/52. Must meet exercise test requirements
MI	Cease for 4/52 After non-ST elevated MI, then 1/52 after angioplasty	Disqualified for 6/52 Relicense after exercise test
Asthma, COPD	Need not notify unless associated with LOC	Need not notify unless associated with LOC
Obstructive sleep apnoea	Cease until controlled	Cease until controlled
Cancer	Need not notify unless brain metastases	Cases assessed on individual basis. Cease for 2 years after lung CA; if no brain metastases, then may drive
CVA	Cease for 1/12	Revocation 12 months after CVA or TIA
Diabetes	Notify DVLA if on tablets or insulin. Advice – warning signs of hypoglycaemia 1, 2, 3 year licence Tablets: retain licence until age 70	IDDM barred Retain licence unless diabetic eye

Condition	Ordinary car licence Group 1	LGV or PCV Group 2
Epilepsy	3 year licence if fit-free for 1 year and only having attacks asleep for 3 years	Fit-free and off treatment for 10 years
Faint (simple)	DVLA need not be notified	No driving restrictions
LOC (unexplained syncope)	Cease for 4/52	Cease for 3/12
LOC with seizure	1 year refusal/revoke markers (tongue bite, incontinence, injury, confused)	5 years refusal/revoke
LOC with no clinical pointers (after investigations)	Refuse/revoke 6/12	Refuse/revoke 1 year
Heart failure	Need not notify	Disqualified if symptomatic Relicense if LVEF > 0.4 and exercise test requirements have been met
Hypertension	Need not notify	Disqualified if SBP consistently 180 or more and/or DBP is 100 mm Hg or more
Migraine	Not drive from onset of warning period	
Psychosis	Cease for 6/12 after inpatient	Suspended licence for 3 years
Vision	6/9 corrected	At least 3/60 uncorrected or 6/9 corrected. Bar if worse than 6/9 in better eye or 6/12 in other eye
Colour blind	Need not notify	Need not notify

General Medical Council – Ethics

Confidentiality

- Ensure anonymity of data; make sure that any identifiable data is edited/changed to reflect anonymity.

- Inform patients prior to making disclosure.

- Seek patient's consent to disclosure of information.

- Ensure that your consultations with patients are private and not overheard.

- Patients may give implied consent to disclosure within the healthcare team.

- Patients have a right of access to their medical records (Data Protection Act 1998).

- Obtain consent to share information with third parties, i.e. social services, other agencies or organisations and offer to show the patient the report. Disclosure without consent (parental or patient) may be justified if failure to do so would expose the patient or others to risk of death or serious harm, i.e. safety of children.

- If you believe a patient to be a victim of neglect or abuse and that patient refuses consent to disclosure, you must give information to the responsible person or statutory agency if disclosure is in the best interest of the patient.

- Disclosure after a patient's death where directions are not clear may then be withheld if it may cause distress to the patient's partner or family or given if it is deemed beneficial. Disclosure may be given: to assist a coroner, procurator fiscal or other officer with an inquest or fatal accident inquiry; to National Confidential Inquiries for education or research (anonymise); on death certificates; to parents of a deceased child, to a partner, close friend or relative; for public interest (Health and Social Care Act 2001); where a person has a right of access to records under the Access to Health Records Act 1990.

- Sending information by fax or e-mail: ensure the fax machines and computer terminals are in secure areas. Anonymise or encrypt electronic data where practicable.

- Access by administrative staff – ensure that administrative data can be accessed separately from clinical information. As administrative staff form part of the healthcare team, sensitive information may be shared with them without the express consent of the patient. Ensure patients are informed who is in the healthcare team and why they may need to access the information. Staff with access to clinical information should understand their duty of confidentiality.

- Disclosure of a sex offender's discharge may be justified if you have good reason to believe that he does not intend to notify the police of his address.

- Unwell doctors – if you think a medical colleague has a drinking problem and is an immediate danger to his/her patients, you must inform the employing authority or the GMC immediately. If you think the problem is under control, you must encourage the colleague to seek help locally from counselling services set up for doctors. You must monitor the colleague's condition and ensure that if this deteriorates, you take immediate action.

Consent

- To investigation and treatment – give details of diagnosis and prognosis, options with benefits and risks, name of the doctor who has overall responsibility, reminder that the patient has the right to change his/her mind or seek a second opinion and details of costs or charges where applicable.

- Withholding information – if the disclosure of information would cause the patient serious harm. Upsetting the patient is not an acceptable exception.

- Patients with fluctuating capacity – document any decisions made while the patient was competent.

- Mentally incapacitated patients – assess the patient's capacity. If the patient refuses any investigation or treatment, you may treat them for any mental disorder under the safeguards of the Mental Health Act 1983. Seek the courts' approval for a non-therapeutic or controversial treatment (contraceptive sterilisation, organ donation, withdrawal of life support from a patient in a persistent vegetative state).

- Advance directives or living wills – you must respect any refusal of treatment given while the patient was competent or if no statement is available, the patient's known wishes should be taken into account.

- Children – at age 16 can be treated as an adult and presumed to have capacity to make decisions. Children under age 16 may give consent if deemed Frazer competent. If a competent child refuses treatment, a legal guardian or the court may authorise investigation or treatment, which is in the child's best interests. If the guardian also refuses treatment, you may seek a ruling from the court. In an emergency, you may treat the child.

Fitness to practise

The Good Medical Practice booklet lists the seven codes of practice as:

1. Providing good clinical care.
2. Maintaining good medical practice – keeping up to date, maintaining your performance.

3. Teaching and training, appraising and assessing.

4. Relationships with patients – obtaining consent, respecting confidentiality, maintaining trust, good communication.

5. Working with colleagues – treat colleagues fairly, working in teams, team leader, sharing information, delegation and referral.

6. Probity – providing information regarding your services, writing reports, giving evidence, signing documents, research, financial and commercial dealings, conflicts of interest.

7. Your health – if your health may put patients at risk.

Groin Lumps

Direct inguinal hernia:

- Lump in superficial inguinal canal that is palpated on the pulp of the finger upon coughing.
- + Cough impulse above inguinal ring.
- Defect in posterior wall of the inguinal canal.
- Medial to internal ring and inferior epigastric vessels.
- Above and medial to pubic tubercle.

Femoral aneurysm:

- Mass with expansile pulsation in line of femoral artery.

Femoral hernia:

- Most common in obese women.
- Below and lateral to pubic tubercle.
- Absence of cough impulse above inguinal ring.

Hydrocoele:

- Can get above scrotal lump between thumb and finger and is translucent.

Incarcerated inguinal hernia:

- Transmits no cough impulse.
- Tense, tender, irreducible.

Indirect inguinal hernia:

- Lump in the superficial inguinal canal palpated on the tip of the finger upon coughing.
- + Cough impulse above inguinal canal.
- Patent process vaginalis.
- Above and medial to pubic tubercle.

Psoas abscess:

- Retrofascial abscess.
- May pass beneath the inguinal ligament and present in the upper part of the femoral triangle.

- Pain on hip extension or internal rotation.

- X-ray shows loss of psoas shadow or mass.

- Soft, compressible, fluctuant mass.

- May elicit fluctuation in parts of abscess above and below inguinal ligament.

Saphena varix:

- Small lump medial to inguinal canal that disappears when lying + associated with varicosities.

- Soft, compressible, expansile dilatation at the top of the saphenous vein.

- Fluid thrill felt if one percusses lower down the saphenous vein.

HIV

As a GP, you will be faced with an increasing HIV population. In South London alone, 1 in 300 residents are infected with the virus. HIV patients are managed at an HIV clinic, with 3-monthly check-ups. These check-ups are to ensure that the viral load is < 30,000 copies/ml and the CD4 count is > 500 cells/mm^3. The CD4 count in a patient without HIV lies between 500 and 1200 cells/mm^3. If the viral load rises above 30,000 copies/ml with the b-DNA test and the CD4 count falls below 500 cells/mm^3 or the CD4 count falls below 350 cells/mm^3, antiviral therapy is advised. A patient with a CD4 count below 200 is at risk for PCP, with up to an 85.5% risk of developing AIDS within 3 years if left untreated. Antiviral therapy can keep the CD4 count high and the viral load down to less than 50 copies/mm^3. In other words, the patient has a good chance of being 'healthy' for more than 10 years before developing AIDS. Of note, the HIV patient will normally have a low Hb, low sodium and high total protein.

In between HIV clinic follow-ups, these patients may present to you, the GP, with the following ailments or queries:

1. **Advice for HIV positive mothers** – with antiviral therapy, close monitoring of antenatal care in a high-risk antenatal clinic and delivery by elective caesarean section, the risk of having an HIV-positive child is 1 in 100.

2. **Cerebral toxoplasmosis** – is treated with sulfadiazine and pyrimethamine.

3. **Dry mouth** – treat with oral nystatin suspension or amphotericin lozenges.

4. **Dry skin** – prescribe Epaderm or E45.

5. **DSS 1500 form for benefits** – complete this form for the patient if the patient has less than 6 months to live.

6. **Oral candidiasis** – this is treated with fluconazole for 2 weeks. Offer a child the suspension form od. An alternative treatment is amphotericin lozenges.

7. **Needlestick injury prophylaxis** – Explain that there is a 1 in 275 risk of acquiring HIV if exposure was to a known needle. Prophylaxis consists of nelfinavir (5 tablets bd), AZT and Combivir to be taken for 1 month. This may also be offered for postcoital rape.

8. *Pneumocystis carinii* **pneumonia prophylaxis** – Septrin (co-trimoxazole). If the patient is allergic to sulfa drugs, offer dapsone or nebulised pentamidine.

9. **Routine blood tests for HIV patients** include CD4 T-cell subset, immunoglobulin, full blood count, amylase and liver function tests.

10. **Shingles** – this is treated with Zovirax (aciclovir) 800 mg five times daily.

11. **Tinea capitis** – prescribe ketoconazole shampoo and offer once a week treatment for prophylaxis.

Some knowledge of the more popularly used antiviral agents is important.

1. **Combivir** (3TC or Epivir) contains AZT and lamivudine. These drugs are NRTIs (nucleoside reverse transcriptase inhibitors) or nucleoside analogues. Side-effects include those associated with AZT as well as diarrhoea and abdominal cramps.

2. **Didanosine** (ddI or Videx) is a NRTI. Side-effects include bloating, diarrhoea, liver problems, nausea, pancreatitis, peripheral neuropathy (burning, numbness or tingling in the hands and/or feet) and vomiting.

3. **Efavirenz** (Sustiva) is a NNRTI (non-nucleoside reverse transcriptase inhibitor). Side-effects include dizziness, liver problems, skin rash and vivid dreams/nightmares.

4. **Nelfinavir** (Viracept) is a protease inhibitor and acts by preventing protease from slicing protein chains into shorter segments necessary for HIV to make new particles. It therefore acts by reducing the number of new active copies of HIV. Side-effects include lipodystrophy, hyperglycaemia, diarrhoea, fatigue, headache, muscle pain and nausea. Monitor the patient's lipid profile and blood glucose.

5. **Nevirapine** (Viramune) is a NNRTI. It is not teratogenic, so may be used in pregnant women. Side-effects include fever, headache, hepatitis, nausea, skin rash and tiredness. Monitor the patient's liver function tests.

6. **Zidovudine** (AZT or Retrovir) is a NRTI. Side-effects include headaches, insomnia, liver problems, muscle pain, nausea, skin rash and vomiting.

Confidentiality, consent and disclosure regarding HIV (GMC's Guidelines on Serious Communicable Diseases)

- You may disclose information to a known sexual contact of a patient with HIV where you have reason to think that the patient has not informed that person and cannot be persuaded to do so. Tell the patient prior to making the disclosure.

- You must disclose information regarding a serious communicable disease to the appropriate authority for notifiable diseases.

- Injuries to health workers (needlestick or exposure to blood/body fluids) – you must obtain patient's consent before undertaking test. If the patient is unconscious, you must wait until he or she regains consciousness to seek consent. If the patient refuses testing or does not regain consciousness in 48 hours, you should consider the severity of the risk. In exceptional circumstances where you have good reason to suspect the patient has HIV for which prophylactic treatment is available, you may test an existing blood sample taken for other purposes. You must be prepared to justify your decision.

- Informing other healthcare professionals – if a patient refuses to allow other healthcare workers to be informed, you must respect this wish except where failure to disclose would put a healthcare worker or other patient at serious risk of death or harm. You should inform the patient, prior to making disclosure.

Hyperlipidaemia Management
British Hypertension Society Guidelines

- Ideal total cholesterol is < 5 mmol/l and ideal LDL cholesterol < 3.0 mmol/l.
- Fasting lipid testing to include TC, triglycerides, HDL and LDL.
- Estimate 10-year CHD risk.
- Secondary causes include alcoholism, anorexia, beta-blockers, biliary cirrhosis, biliary obstruction, chronic renal failure, corticosteroids, diabetes, nephrotic syndrome, pregnancy, retinoids and thiazides.
- Step 1 diet: total fat < 35% of calories (< 10% saturated fat) and cholesterol < 300 mg.
- Step 2 diet: total fat < 25% of calories (< 7% saturated fat) and cholesterol < 300 mg.

Total cholesterol	10-year CHD risk	Measures	Further action
< 5.0	< 15%	Lifestyle advice	Reassess in 5 years
	≥ 15%	Lifestyle advice Lipoprotein analysis Correct secondary causes	Reassess annually
≥ 5.0	< 15%	Correct secondary causes Trial of lipid-lowering diet Check effect at 1 and 3 months	Refer to dietitian Reassess annually once stable
	≥ 15%	Lipoprotein analysis Correct secondary causes Trial of lipid-lowering diet If step 1 diet fails, try step 2 diet	If diet fails, add statin. Fibrates if both TC and TG are raised. Nicotinic acid and bile sequestrants are second line adjuncts
Familial dyslipidaemia			Refer to specialist for treatment regardless of CHD risk

For triglycerides:

- < 2.3 mmol/l, no treatment.
- > 2.3 mmol/l with normal TC or moderately raised TC, correct secondary cause and start trial of lipid-lowering diet for 6 months. If fails, commence nicotinic acid or fibrate and monitor every 3 months.
- If > 4.5 mmol/l refer to specialist lipid clinic as patients are at risk of acute pancreatitis.

Hypertension Management

Blood pressure	SBP (mm Hg)	DBP (mm Hg)
Optimal	< 120	< 80
Normal	< 130	< 85
High normal	130–139	85–89
Grade 1 (mild hypertension)	140–159	90–99
Grade 2 (moderate)	160–179	100–109
Grade 3 (severe)	≥ 180	≥ 110
Isolated systolic hypertension	140–159 (grade 1)	< 90
Isolated systolic hypertension	≥ 160 (grade 2)	< 90

Blood pressure (mm Hg)	Recommended action (advise all patients re lifestyle measures)
< 130/85	Reassess in 5 years
< 130–139/85–89	Reassess annually
140–159/90–99	Re-measure monthly if 10-year CHD risk < 20% and no target organ damage, no CV complications and no diabetes. Observe and reassess CHD risk annually
140–159/90–99	If the 10-year CHD risk is ≥ 20%, target organ damage, CV complications or diabetes, confirm over 12 weeks, then treat
160–179/100–109	Re-measure weekly if 10-year CHD risk is < 20% and no target organ damage, no CV complications and no diabetes. Treat if BP remains at this level over 4–12 weeks
160–179/100–109	If the 10-year CHD risk is ≥ 20%, target organ damage, CV complications or diabetes, confirm over 3–4 weeks, then treat if BP remains at this level
≥ 160/100	Regardless of 10-year CHD risk, confirm over 1–2 weeks, then treat
> 180/110	Regardless of 10-year CHD risk, confirm over 1–2 weeks, then treat. If malignant hypertension or hypertensive emergency, admit immediately

Evaluation of hypertensive patients:

- Measure sitting BP every 5 years.
- Check standing BPs in elderly or diabetic patients at least at the initial estimation.
- Take the mean of at least two readings.
- Use ambulatory blood pressure monitoring for:
  - determining the efficacy of drug treatment over 24 hours
  - diagnosis and treatment of hypertension in pregnancy
  - evaluation of drug-resistant hypertension
  - nocturnal hypertension
  - unusual variability of BP
  - 'white-coat' hypertension
- Estimate 10-year CHD risk:
- Major risk factors include cardiovascular disease, coronary heart disease risk > 20%, diabetes and target organ damage. Other risk factors include age, family history, male sex, total cholesterol : HDL ratio and smoking.

Investigations:

- ECG.
- Fasting blood glucose.
- Fasting blood lipid profile (TC, HDL, TG).
- Serum creatinine and electrolytes.
- Urine strip test for protein and blood.

Causes of hypertension:

- Coarctation (radiofemoral delay or weak femoral pulses).
- Conn's syndrome (hypokalaemia, muscle weakness, polyuria, tetany).
- Cushing's disease.
- Drugs (combined oral contraceptives, liquorice, NSAIDs, steroids, sympathomimetics).
- Phaeochromocytoma (paroxysmal symptoms).
- Renal disease (proteinuria or haematuria, family history, palpable kidney (hydronephrosis, neoplasm or polycystic)).
- Renovascular disease (abdominal or loin bruit).

Target organ damage or complications:

- Angina, CABG/angioplasty, heart failure, LVH or left ventricular strain on ECG, MI.
- Carotid bruits, dementia, stroke and transient ischaemic attack.

- Fundal haemorrhages, papilloedema.
- Peripheral vascular disease.
- Proteinuria, renal impairment.

Lifestyle measures:

- Reduce the intake of total and saturated fat.
- Reduce salt (< 6 g NaCl/day or 100 mmol/day)
- Reduce environmental stress, and weight if BMI > 25.
- Advise five portions/day of fruit and vegetables per day.
- Stop smoking.
- Take up regular aerobic exercise for ≥ 30 minutes a day at least 3 times a week.
- Limit weekly alcohol intake to < 21 units (men) and < 14 units (women).

Treatment:

	Non-black or < 55 years	**Black or > 55 years**
Step 1:	ACEI/angiotensin II antagonist (A) or beta-blocker (B))	calcium channel blocker (C) or thiazide diuretic (D)
Step 2:	A (or B) + (C or D)	
Step 3:	A (or B) + C + D	
Step 4:	A + B + C + D or add alpha-blocker or spironolactone or other diuretic	

Add statin if CHD risk ≥ 20% and total cholesterol ≥ 3.5 mmol/l.

Add aspirin 75 mg daily if age ≥ 50 years, with BP < 150/90 mm Hg and target organ damage, diabetes or 10-year CV risk ≥ 20%.

Refer to specialist:

- Malignant hypertension/emergency (accelerated hypertension with grade III–IV retinopathy).
- Severe hypertension > 220/120 mm Hg.
- Impending complications of LVF, TIA, etc.
- Hypertension in a patient < 20 years or needing treatment in a patient < 30 years.
- Investigation of underlying secondary causes.
- Resistance to multidrug regimen (≥ 3 drugs).
- Evaluation of therapeutic problems (multiple drug intolerance, contraindications, non-compliance).
- White-coat hypertension, pregnancy and variable BP.

Drug treatment of hypertension: WHO guidelines

Class of drug	Indications	Contraindications
ACEI	CHF, LVF, after MI, diabetic nephropathy	Hyperkalaemia, bilateral renal artery stenosis
Alpha-blockers	BPH, glucose intolerance	Orthostatic hypotension
Angiotensin II antagonists	ACEI cough	CHF, bilateral renal artery stenosis, ↑K
Beta-blockers	After MI, angina, tachyarrhythmias	CHF, asthma, COPD, heart block, diabetes
Calcium antagonists	Angina, elderly, systolic hypertension	Grade 2 or 3 heart block with verapamil or diltiazem
Diuretics	CHF, elderly, systolic hypertension	Gout

Hypertension and Hyperlipidaemia in Type 2 Diabetes
NICE Guidelines October 2002

Summary of recommendations:

- Annual estimate of heart disease risk with BP and blood lipid levels.

- If BP $\geq$ 140/80, and < 15% 10-year coronary event risk, then offer advice on lifestyle changes.

- If BP $\geq$ 140/80, and > 15% 10-year coronary event risk, then offer treatment.

- If BP $\geq$ 160/100, offer treatment to reduce BP to < 140/80.

- If BP $\geq$ 140/80 and albumin or protein in urine, then offer treatment to lower BP to 135/75 or lower.

- For people with a history of cardiovascular disease, give 75 mg aspirin a day.

- If total cholesterol level is $\geq$ 5.0 mmol/l or a triglyceride level of 2.3 mmol/l or more, then exclude secondary causes, ensure blood glucose levels are well controlled, offer lifestyle advice, etc. Aim to reduce total cholesterol to below 5 mmol/l or to 75–80% of the level prior to treatment or to reduce LDL-C to below 3 mmol/l or to 70% of the level prior to treatment, whichever is lower.

Medical Certificates

Self-certificate (SC1) Patients who are not eligible for statutory sick pay but who wish to claim for incapacity benefit. Certifies for first 7 days of illness

Self-certificate (SC2) As SC1 but for statutory sick pay. Forms may be obtained from the surgery, employer or local Jobcentre Plus

Med3 Filled in by GP who is familiar with the patient and the period of incapacity is > 7 days. Closed certificate – gives a specific date of return if illness is < 14 days. Open certificate – specifies a period of time, e.g. 13 weeks for nervous debility. Patient will need a fitness to work certificate to return to work. Patient must be seen within 1 day of signing. Certificate may not be backdated

Med4 After 28 weeks' incapacity; patient is sent form IB50 and asked for med4 from GP. The Department of Works and Pensions may ask for further medical examination

Med5 On basis of recent other doctor's report (< 1 month), the doctor may sign med5 on patient's behalf; not to exceed a forward period of > 1 month; the patient returns to work without receiving a med3; backdating certificate if condition is ongoing and the patient was not seen within 1 day of illness

Med6 A vague diagnosis is put on the form if it is deemed to be harmful to the patient or detrimental for the employer to know the true diagnosis; the med6 requests the Jobcentre Plus to send an additional form for more details

RM7 Form sent to Jobcentre Plus asking them to review patient sooner than would otherwise be done if doubt about disability

DS1500 Terminal illness, not expected to live longer than 6 months

Mental Health Act 1983

Section 2	Admit for ASSESSMENT, compulsory to hospital, up to 28 days, not renewable, requires two doctors (one approved under section 12 and one GP), application for admission by social worker or nearest relative (spouse, offspring, parent)
Section 3	Admit for TREATMENT, compulsory to hospital, up to 6 months, has diagnosis, requires two doctors (one section 12 and one GP), application for admission by social worker or nearest relative
Section 4	EMERGENCY admission, compulsory to hospital, 72 hours, not renewable, GP seen patient in last 24 hours, requires one doctor if 'urgent necessity' and social worker or nearest relative, change to section 2 later
Section 5	DETAIN INPATIENT by one doctor in emergency only or by nurse in hospital, 72 hours. If doctor is not a psychiatrist, he or she must act in person to contact a psychiatrist; section 2 or 3 can be considered
Section 7	Appropriate for GUARDIANSHIP (reception into)
Section 12	Used to approve doctors recognised as having special expertise in mental health
Section 115	Right of entry into premises by social worker
Section 135	Police right of entry into premises to remove patient to place of safety under a magistrate's warrant
Section 136	Police right to remove patient from public place to place of safety (prison cell or hospital) for 72 hours to allow medical examination

Methods/Study Designs

Design of study

Cross-sectional surveys:

- **Prevalence** studies, descriptive study which provides a **snapshot** of the population in question.

- The presence or absence of disease can be assessed and compared with age, sex or body weight.

- **Cannot assess incidence of exact timing of exposure or cause or effect.**

- Example: use of Mirena (intrauterine progestogen-only contraceptive) by female doctors – current use percentage vs age group; random postal questionnaire between 1990 and 1995.

Case-control studies:

- Case (subjects with disease) and controls (same population as cases but no disease).

- **Retrospective** studies.

- Look for **exposure** or presence of factor **association not causation.**

- Assess by questionnaire, interviews or medical records.

- Investigate hypothesis and may be followed up by cohort or intervention studies.

- **Cannot calculate incidence of disease, true relative risk, attributable risk.**

- **Can calculate odds ratio** (estimate of relative risk) if incidence of disease in general population < 5%, control group representative of general population, and cases + controls free from selection bias.

- Pros – **small number of subjects**, can assess **rare** conditions, **quick + cheap, multiple exposures.**

- Cons: **problems of bias**, retrospective (recall-bias), hard to establish causal relationship, hard to select controls.

- Example: lung CA in shipyard workers – cases vs controls (relatives).

Cohort studies:

- **Prospective** (looking ahead), for **rare exposures and several outcomes** may be studied.

- Pros – **can calculate incidence directly, relative risk, attributable risk.**

- Selection bias is less likely.
- Several exposures can be evaluated from exposures to same agent.
- Cons – hard to interpret causal relationships, expensive as large population studied over long time, loss of follow-up can affect validity.
- Example: study starts 1980s and ends 20 years later, series of observations made on subjects.

Randomised controlled trials (clinical):

- Intervention studies prompted by findings of case-control, cohort or cross-sectional survey.
- Intervention (treated) group vs control group allocated in a random manner.
- Gives best evidence of cause + effect.
- Example: treatment with interferon for MS.

Other terminology used

Conclusions:

- Difference between general population and sample study group due to chance sampling variation, study biases, confounding factors or true difference.

Null hypothesis:

- There is no difference between the two groups; the intervention has no effect.

Test of statistical significance:

- Based on null hypothesis; examples: *t*-test, chi-squared.

ρ value:

- Probability of this result occurring by chance, if null hypothesis is true.
- ρ value < 0.05 indicates statistical significance, < 1/20 due to chance.
- ρ value irrelevant if study + biases, confounding factors, small sample size.

Confidence interval:

- % probability that true value lies within the confidence limits.
- Example: 95% CI = 95% chance true value lies within stated limits or 5% chance lies outside.
- Desire narrow CI less chance of variability in sample and greater certainty.

Relative risk:

- Results of cohort studies; ratio of disease incidence in exposed vs non-exposed.

- RR = 1 (no association between exposure + outcome); example: RR for cholelithiasis with obesity = 2 (0.8 – 2.7) 95% CI.

Notifiable Diseases
(under the Public Health Act of 1984 and Public Health Regulations 1988)

anthrax

cholera

diphtheria

dysentery (amoebic or bacillary)

encephalitis

food poisoning (suspected or proven)

lassa fever

leprosy

leptospirosis

malaria

Marburg disease

measles

meningitis

mumps

ophthalmia neonatorum

paratyphoid A or B

plague

polio

rabies

relapsing fever

rubella

scarlet fever

smallpox

tetanus

tuberculosis

typhoid fever

typhus fever

viral haemorrhagic fever

viral hepatitis

whooping cough

yellow fever

Obstetrics

Abortion   termination of pregnancy, spontaneous or induced, prior to 24 weeks' gestation

Incomplete abortion   PV bleed in early pregnancy associated with passage of products of conception and an open cervical os

Inevitable abortion   PV bleed in early pregnancy associated with an open cervical os and no passage of products of conception

Missed abortion   small for dates uterus with closed cervical os; fetal death

Septic abortion   any type of abortion that becomes infected

Threatened abortion   PV spotting in early pregnancy with a closed cervical os and no passage of products of conception

Placenta abruptio   antepartum PV bleed after 24 weeks' gestation associated with lower abdominal pain due to separation of the placenta before delivery of the infant

Placenta praevia   antepartum painless recurrent PV bleed after 24 weeks' gestation due to a low-lying placenta; vaginal examination must not be performed if suspect praevia

Postpartum haemorrhage   **Primary** – blood loss $\geq$ 500 ml within 24 hours of delivery

                                   Secondary – blood loss $\geq$ 500 ml after the first 24 hours; usually due to infection or retained products of conception

Osteoporosis

- Reduced bone mass and microarchitectural deterioration of bone.
- WHO definition: hip or spine bone density T score ≤ -2.5.
- Susceptible to fractures in hips (women > 75 years), vertebrae (associated with steroid use so give osteoporosis protection) and wrists (Colles in women > 65 years).
- Postmenopausal women lose 2% per year in bone mass for the first 8 years and then 1% per year. By age 80, a woman will have lost 30–40% of her bone mass.

Risk factors:

- Previous fracture from minor fall.
- Females who have a natural or early surgical menopause before age 45.
- Premenopausal amenorrhoea > 6 months not due to pregnancy.
- Alcoholism.
- Family history of osteoporosis (doubles risk).
- Liver disease.
- Malabsorption.
- Male hypogonadism.
- Prolonged bedrest.
- Rheumatoid arthritis (on systemic steroids).
- Smoking.
- Steroid use in the following conditions: (> 7.5 mg prednisolone per day for > 3 months, i.e. rheumatoid arthritis), polymyalgia rheumatica (50 mg prednisolone daily and tapered over 18 months), asthma, COPD (short bursts of steroids do not increase risk), ulcerative colitis.
- Thyroid disease.
- Suggest investigate risk factors with blood tests: TFTs, vitamin B level and ESR.
- Fat is protective.

Prevention:

- Avoid exercise-related amenorrhoea.
- Give all women > 75 years Calcichew D3 Forte one tablet a day or regular Calcichew two tablets a day.

- Limit alcohol intake.
- Maintain recommended daily intake of 700 mg calcium and 400 IU vitamin D (90% from the sun). Postmenopausal women require 1.5 g of calcium.
- Regular weight-bearing exercise.
- Smoking cessation.

Hip fracture:

- 20% of patients with hip fractures die within a year after this major operation (National Service Framework 2001).
- 50% lose their independence and need to rely on a stick or nursing home placement (National Service Framework 2001).
- 60% are unable to walk independently to 12 metres (NICE 2000).
- Average age of patient at risk is 80 years.

Vertebral fractures:

- Often painless.
- First sign may be shrinkage or loss of inches in height, i.e. dowager's hump.
- Elicit pain by asking patient to sneeze or cough and if the pain radiates around the ribs and waist to the front, highly suspicious of vertebral fracture.

Medication:

- Bisphosphonates – personal favourite is the once a week second generation bisphosphonate alendronate (Fosamax); give with Calcichew D3 Forte; protective against both hip and vertebral fractures. Alternative is risedronate which increases bone density and is purported to decrease incidence of hip fractures by 40%.
- Raloxifene – drug of choice for patients with a history of breast CA, family history or MI. A synthetic oestrogen receptor modulator. MORE (multiple outcomes of raloxifene) double-blinded placebo-controlled trial published in JAMA, 1999, showed risk reduction of both breast cancer and vertebral fractures with raloxifene.

Refer:

- Kyphosis or loss in height.
- Multiple risk factors.
- Osteopenia on x-ray.
- Osteoporosis with or without fracture.
- Prolonged use of steroids > 3 months.

Rheumatoid Arthritis

- Age of onset – 20–35 years. Females have three times greater risk than males.
- Symmetrical arthritis involving MCP, MTP, PIP and wrists.
- Hallmark symptoms: early morning stiffness.
- Fatigue.

Investigations:

- FBC.
- ESR.
- CRP (very sensitive to inflammation and is superior to ESR for diagnosing polymyalgia rheumatica).
- Rheumatoid factor (positive in 70%; 30% are normal with a positive RF and 30% are false negatives).
- Biochemistry.

Associated with poor prognosis:

- Elderly.
- Female.
- High ESR, CRP, alkaline phosphatase and platelets.
- Multiple affected joints at onset.
- Positive rheumatoid factor – the higher the worse the prognosis.
- Systemic involvement (iritis, pleural effusion and vasculitis).

Treatment:

- Early referral to rheumatologist
- Aggressive first-line treatment with methotrexate + Salazopyrin (sulfasalazine) + hydroxychloroquine +/− prednisolone. Drug combinations are used to switch the disease off and prevent erosions.
- Newer agents (disease-modifying drugs) such as infliximab (injections per 2 months) and etanercept are expensive and cost £10 000 a year.

Screening Programme

- **Important** condition.

- **Acceptable** treatment for the disease.

- **Adequate** treatment and diagnostic facilities available.

- **Recognisable** latent or early symptomatic stage.

- **Opinions** on who to treat are agreed.

- **Guaranteed** safety and reliability of test.

- **Examination** acceptable to patient.

- **Natural history of disease** is known.

- **Inexpensive** and simple test suitable.

- **Continuous** repeated at intervals determined by natural history of disease.

Statistics

Sick and fit studies

		Disease	
		+	−
Exposure/test	+	A	B
	−	C	D

Sensitivity = proportion of true positives (TP) correctly identified by test = A/A+C (SICK)

Specificity = proportion of true negatives (TN) correctly identified by test = D/B+D (FIT)

Positive predictive value (PPV) = proportion of patients with positive test correctly identified as diseased = A/A+B

Negative predictive value (NPV) = proportion of patients with negative test correctly identified as disease-free = D/C+D

Example 1

Population of 100, prevalence of disease is 1% = 1 with disease, 99 without disease. The test has 100% sensitivity and 95% specificity:

		Disease		
		+	−	
Test	+	1	5	6
	−	0	94	94
		1	99	100
		TP	TN	total population

PPV = 1/6 = 17%
NPV = 94/94= 100%

Example 2

Population of 500 in a small town in China. 100 inhabitants have AIDS. 80/100 with the disease test positive correctly; 50 who have no disease test positive.

		Disease		
		+	−	
Test	+	80	50	= 130
	−	20	350	= 370
		100	400	500
		TP	TN	total population

Prevalence of disease is $100/500 = 20\%$
Sensitivity of test $= 80/100 = 80\%$
Specificity of test $= 350/400 = 87.5\%$
PPV $= 80/130 = 62\%$
NPV $= 350/370 = 95\%$

Example 3

Mammography screening test. Specificity 80%, sensitivity 90%. Population of 1000 females aged 50–65 with prevalence of breast CA 10%.

PPV $= 90/270 = 33\%$
NPV $= 720/730 = 99\%$

Cohort studies

Relative risk:

Disease rate in exposed group divided by disease rate in non-exposed group; incidence of disease in exposed (exp) population divided by incidence of disease in non-exposed (NE) population.

Division:

$$\frac{A}{A+B} \div \frac{C}{C+D} = \frac{\text{dis in exp}}{\text{dis in exp} + \text{no dis in exp}} \div \frac{+ \text{dis in NE}}{+ \text{dis in NE} + \text{no dis in NE}}$$

i.e. relative risk $= 1 =$ exposure is not associated with an increased or decreased risk of disease; i.e. no effect on the disease.

Attributable risk:

Excess risk (or outcome) attributable to a given exposure.

Subtract:

$$\frac{A}{A+B} - \frac{C}{C+D} = \frac{\text{dis in exp}}{\text{dis in exp} + \text{no dis in exp}} - \frac{+ \text{dis in NE}}{+ \text{dis in NE} + \text{no dis in NE}}$$

Case-control studies

Exposure rate for cases: $\quad \dfrac{A}{A+C} = \dfrac{\text{dis in exp}}{\text{dis in exp} + \text{dis in NE}}$

Exposure rate for controls: $\quad \dfrac{B}{B+D} = \dfrac{\text{no dis in exp}}{\text{no dis in exp} + \text{no dis in NE}}$

Odds ratio is the estimate of relative risk:

$$\frac{A \times (C+D)}{C \times (A+B)} = \frac{\text{dis in exp} \times (\text{dis in NE} + \text{no dis in NE})}{\text{dis in NE} \times (\text{dis in exp} + \text{no dis in exp})} \sim \frac{A \times D}{C \times B}$$

Example 4

		DVT		
		+	–	
Pill use	+	A=100	B=200	100/300 women using pill get DVT (dis)
	–	C = 200	D = 800	200/1000 controls not on pill get DVT
		$\overline{300}$	$\overline{1000}$	

$$\text{Odds ratio} = \frac{A \times D}{C \times B} = \frac{100 \times 800}{200 \times 200} = 2 = \text{pill users have a two times higher risk of DVT}$$

Cohort

Example 5

100 in 1000 female smokers at risk of cervical CA. 60 in 1000 female non-smokers at risk of cervical CA.

		Disease (cervical CA)		
		+	–	
Exposed to tobacco	+	100	900	1000
	–	60	940	1000

- Absolute risk (incidence) in general female population
$$= 60/1000 = 6 \text{ in } 100 = 1 \text{ in } 17$$

- Relative risk (incidence in exp population
÷ incidence in NE population) = $\dfrac{100}{1000} \div \dfrac{60}{1000} = 1.67$

- Attributable risk (incidence in exposed population – incidence in NE population) $= \dfrac{100}{1000} - \dfrac{60}{1000} = \dfrac{40}{1000} = 0.04$

Example 6

Smoking increases risk of lung CA by 40%. Smoking decreases risk of Parkinson's disease by 20%.

- Relative risk of lung CA in smokers vs nonsmokers? $1 + (40\% \text{ of } 1) = 1.4$

- Relative risk of PD in smokers vs nonsmokers? $1 - (20\% \text{ of } 1) = 0.8$

NNT (numbers needed to treat)

Definition:

- Number of individuals who need to be treated to achieve one desired outcome.

- Reciprocal of the reduction in absolute risk (absolute risk reduction or ARR).

- **1/ARR%.**

- Depends on prevalence of given disease, i.e. high AR or incidence of heart disease: low NNT to prevent one death.

ARR = proportion of treated group – proportion of controls
with desired outcome with desired outcome

ARR% = % treated group with desired – % controls with desired
outcome outcome

Example 7

% giving up smoking in treated group with amfebutamone
$$= 10/100 = 10\%$$

% giving up smoking in control group $= 12/200 = 6\%$

ARR% = 10% – 6% = 4%

NNT = 1/ARR% = 1/4% = 25 people needed to be given bupropion to cause 1 person to quit.

Stroke Secondary Prevention

Royal College of Physicians National Clinical Guidelines 2002

1. Hypertension:

- All patients should have their BP checked, and hypertension persisting for more than 1 month should be treated. The BHS optimal BP targets are SBP < 140 mm Hg and DBP < 85 mm Hg with a minimal acceptable BP of < 150/< 90 mm Hg. For diabetic patients, the target is 140/85.

- Further reduction should be considered using a combination of long-acting ACE inhibitors (i.e. perindopril or ramipril) and a thiazide diuretic (i.e. indapamide).

2. Antiplatelet therapy:

- All patients with ischaemic stroke who are not on anticoagulation should be taking aspirin 75–325 mg daily or clopidogrel or a combination of low-dose aspirin and dipyridamole modified release. Patients with aspirin intolerance should take clopidogrel 75 mg daily or dipyridamole MR 200 mg daily.

3. Anticoagulation:

- Should not be used after TIAs or minor strokes unless suspect cardiac embolism.

- Should not be started until brain imaging has excluded haemorrhage and 14 days have passed from the onset of an ischaemic stroke.

- Should be started in every patient in atrial fibrillation (non-valvular and valvular) unless contraindicated.

- Should be considered for all patients who have ischaemic stroke associated with mitral valve disease, prosthetic heart valves or within 3 months of an MI.

4. Carotid endarterectomy:

- Any patient with a carotid artery area stroke, and minor or absent residual disability, should be considered for carotid endarterectomy.

- Carotid ultrasound should be performed on candidates who would be considered for carotid endarterectomy. Magnetic resonance angiography is a reasonable alternative.

- Should be considered where the carotid stenosis is > 70%.

- Should only be undertaken by a specialist surgeon with a proven low complication rate.

- Carotid angioplasty or stenting is an alternative to surgery but should only be carried out in centres with a proven low complication rate.

5. Lifestyle management:

- All patients should be assessed for other vascular risk factors and advised and treated appropriately.

- All patients should be given appropriate advice on lifestyle factors (avoid added salt and excess alcohol, diet, maintaining ideal weight, regular exercise, smoking cessation).

6. Lipids:

- Statin therapy should be considered for all patients with a history of ischaemic heart disease and a cholesterol of > 5 mmol/l following stroke.

Urinary Incontinence

History	length of time, frequency, amount of leakage, fluid intake, present management and impact on lifestyle
Examination	abdomen, PR, PV, relevant neurological examination
Investigation	frequency/volume chart, residual urine estimation (scan or in/out catheterisation), urine dipstick/MSU

Stress incontinence

Symptoms	leaking with coughing, exercise or laughing
Aetiology	urethral sphincter incompetence, pelvic floor weakness
Treatment	pelvic floor exercises, urethral appliances, surgery
Referral	continence specialist nurse, physiotherapist, uro-gynaecologist, urologist

Detrusor overactivity

Symptoms	urgency, frequency (> 7/24 hours), urge incontinence
Aetiology	idiopathic, secondary to neurological disease (multiple sclerosis), atrophic urethritis/vaginitis, bladder calculus refer to surgeons, cystitis, UTI treat with antibiotics

Treatment for idiopathic/neurological
check residual volume, advice on fluid intake, bladder retraining programme, anticholinergic drugs

Treatment for atrophic urethritis/vaginitis
topical oestrogen replacement or systemic HRT

Bladder outlet obstruction

Symptoms	voiding inefficiency, continual dribbling, weak flow, hesitancy, incomplete voiding, intermittent stream, straining to void

Aetiology	prostate hypertrophy, urethral stricture, faecal impaction
Treatment	refer to prostate assessment clinic, urologist

Detrusor failure

Symptoms	voiding inefficiency (see above)
Aetiology	secondary to neurological disease
Treatment	clean intermittent catheterisation if postmicturition residual > 150 ml
Referral	continence specialist nurse, specialist continence service
Confounding factors	alpha-adrenoreceptor blockers, anticholinergics, calcium channel blockers, diuretics, sedatives

Vaginal Discharge

Bacterial vaginosis
(Gardnerella vaginalis)

gram-negative rod; fishy odour, bubble-bath, douching, stringy grey-yellow raw-egg-white discharge, not sexually transmitted, salt and pepper appearance on microscopy; px metronidazole 400 mg bd for 5 days

Chlamydia trachomatis

obligate intracellular parasite; STD, may be asymptomatic, mucopurulent cervicitis, contact bleeding; endocervical swab; cause of infertility, ectopic pregnancy, PID; px doxycycline 100 mg bd for 1 week or azithromycin 1 g STAT

Gonorrhoea

Gram-negative diplococcus; STD, purulent yellow-green discharge, HVS, urethral, rectal swabs; px ciprofloxacin 500 mg STAT; reculture 3–7 days after treatment; contact tracing

PID

px cipro STAT + doxycycline 100 mg bd for 2 weeks + metronidazole 400 mg bd for 5 days

Thrush
(candidiasis)

white cheesy discharge, pruritus vulvae, superficial dyspareunia; predisposing factors (Addison's or Cushing's disease, broad-spectrum antibiotics, DM, immunosuppression, pregnancy, steroids); px clotrimazole pessary and cream

Trichomonas vaginalis

STD, mucopurulent, yellow, frothy discharge; strawberry-red cervix; flagellate trophozoite protozoa; px metronidazole 400 mg bd for 5 days